A WOMAN DOCTOR'S GUIDE TO PMS

A WOMAN DOCTOR'S GUIDE TO PMS

Essential Facts and
Up-to-the-Minute Information on
Premenstrual Syndrome

By

Andrea J. Rapkin, M.D., F.A.C.O.G.

with

Diana Tonnessen

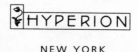

HYPERION

NEW YORK

LIBRARY OF CONGRESS CATALOGING-IN-PUBLICATION DATA

Rapkin, Andrea J.
    A woman doctor's guide to PMS : essential facts and up-to-the-minute
information on premenstrual syndrome / Andrea J. Rapkin and
Diana Tonnessen.
        p. cm.
    ISBN 1-56282-810-X
    1. Premenstrual syndrome—Popular works. I. Tonnessen, Diana.
II. Title.
    [DNLM: 1. Premenstrual Syndrome—diagnosis. 2. Premenstrual
Syndrome—therapy.   WP 560 R218w 1994]
RG165.R357 1994
618.1'72—dc20
DNLM/DLC   94-10992
                                                                  CIP

FIRST EDITION

10 9 8 7 6 5 4 3 2 1

Many thanks to Barbara Lowenstein,
Eileen Fallon, and Nancy Friedman

—Diana Tonnessen

CREDITS

CONTENTS

LIST OF
ILLUSTRATIONS

A WOMAN
DOCTOR'S
GUIDE TO
PMS

CHAPTER 1

PMS: FACT VERSUS FICTION

For years, you've put "mind over matter," telling yourself that if you keep a stiff upper lip, you *can* conquer the crying jags and cravings for peanut M&Ms that occasionally overwhelm you. But for some reason, your resolve starts to crumble about a week before your period. . .

You can tell when your period is approaching because your pants don't fit and your breasts become sore. But it's nothing that an over-the-counter water pill can't help. . .

The magnitude of the fight you had with your husband last night was as bewildering to him as it was to you. It was as though a part of you stood by helpless, saying "what's the big deal? So he forgot to take out the garbage?" while another part of you railed on, unable to contain your rage. You'd like to cuddle up to your husband and give him a big hug, but instead you hide behind a book all day, deliberately avoiding him for fear of picking another fight. . .

You've noticed that even your children have started tiptoeing around, trying "not to upset Mom when she's having one of her bad days," which, come to think of it, is usually about once a month. . .

If any of these scenarios sound familiar to you, you're not alone. An estimated 30 to 40 percent of all women at some point in their reproductive years experience physical and emotional symptoms just prior to menstruation that are serious enough to cause distress, what many of us refer to as *premen-*

strual syndrome, or PMS. From 5 to 10 percent of these women suffer debilitating symptoms that seriously interfere with their lives—Jekyll-and-Hyde mood swings, feelings of hopelessness and despair, irritability, a seemingly insatiable appetite for sweets, pounding headaches, bloating and breast tenderness, crushing fatigue, and sometimes even suicidal thoughts. For most women, symptoms clear up like clockwork a day or two after the onset of menstruation—until the following month.

As common as these symptoms are, the syndrome itself is as baffling as ever. There are no clear-cut diagnostic tests that can tell you definitively whether you have PMS. For this reason, no one is really certain just how widespread the condition is. Complicating matters even further is the fact that premenstrual symptoms vary from woman to woman and may even affect the same woman differently at different times in her life.

Even the experts don't agree on the nature of the disorder; that is, whether PMS has psychological or physical roots. Adding to the confusion are studies—often poorly designed—suggesting that such treatments as vitamin B_6, evening primrose oil, L-tryptophan or over-the-counter diuretics can help "cure" PMS. Some of these studies make headlines in the mass media, but their shortcomings are often glossed over or ignored altogether.

If you're like most women, you may have brushed off your symptoms as simply an annoying part of being a woman. Or perhaps you're too embarrassed even to mention them to your doctor for fear of being told that your problem is "all in your head." Chances are good you spend quite a bit of time and energy covering up your symptoms, overcompensating for what you perceive to be poor performance on the job (or sometimes just calling in sick), or isolating yourself from your husband and children to protect them from your depression or irritability. In your more desperate moments, you may have even tried a few of the above-mentioned alternative remedies, such as vitamin B_6, or L-tryptophan. After all, you reason, what harm could come of it?

Unfortunately, this kind of thinking can be dangerous. In fact, sales of the nutritional supplement L-tryptophan were banned by the United States Food and Drug Administration in 1990 after a contaminated batch of supplements manufactured in Japan was associated with a serious, sometimes fatal blood disorder known as *eosinophilia myalgia syndrome*. Even such seemingly "safe" treatments as vitamin B_6 and over-the-counter diuretics can have bothersome and potentially harmful side effects. When taken in large doses (more than 100 mg per day—a dosage frequently recommended for women with PMS), vitamin B_6 can cause a tingling sensation in the hands and feet, an unsteady gait, and other symptoms associated with *sensory neuropathy*, a type of nerve damage. Over-the-counter diuretics can have a rebound effect, causing you to retain even more fluid when you stop taking them.

Perhaps even more worrisome is that the fear and confusion surrounding PMS may keep you from getting an accurate diagnosis and appropriate treatment, which simply prolongs your suffering and undermines your self-esteem. Here's a look at some of the fictions and half-truths that many people associate with PMS. Have any of these beliefs kept you from taking control of your situation?

FICTION: It's all in your head.

FACT: It's easy for people who don't suffer from premenstrual syndrome (and even some doctors) to toss it off as "all in your head," particularly when researchers still don't know the exact causes of PMS. But for you, the symptoms are undeniably real.

Although much remains to be learned about the disorder, research over the past several years has established premenstrual syndrome as a very real medical condition with identifiable symptoms, specific criteria for making a diagnosis, and a variety of effective treatment approaches.

FICTION: PMS isn't all that serious; it affects you only one week out of the month.

FACT: Depending on the severity of your symptoms, PMS can color every aspect of your life, undermining your relationship with your husband or "significant other," your children and co-workers, and eroding your self esteem—even when it's not "that time of the month." Even if premenstrual symptoms cause you to miss work or cancel social engagements just one day out of the month, over the years that one day can add up to weeks or even months. That's a sizable chunk of your life to be missing out on. And that's why you owe it to yourself to get professional help for your PMS.

FICTION: Menstruation and premenstrual tension affect a woman's ability to think clearly, and women can't function as well as usual just before or during their periods.

FACT: It's this kind of thinking that causes many women to ignore or try to hide their symptoms—even from other women. No one wants to be fired from her job, kept from getting a promotion, or barred from public office—or to be held responsible for holding other women back—because she has PMS. Rest assured that while you may not *feel* as though you are giving your all when you are experiencing breast tenderness, bloating, food cravings, mood swings or other premenstrual symptoms, *almost 50 years of research has shown no* *consistent, demonstrable effect of the menstrual cycle on work or academic performance.* So let your boss and other women in on the good news.

FICTION: PMS is just an excuse for some women who have a tendency to be overemotional.

FACT: PMS is not an excuse; it's a medical condition that causes certain symptoms, including mood swings, blue moods, and feelings of hopelessness and despair. You should be aware, however, that PMS isn't always the only cause of these symptoms. In fact, many women who seek treatment for PMS actually suffer from such psychological disorders as anxiety and depression. Fortunately, these are some of the most common and easily treated emotional problems. So whatever the cause of being "overemotional," there's no excuse for not getting help.

FICTION: PMS is a "woman's problem."

FACT: In reality, premenstrual changes are only one of a number of cyclic changes in mood and behavior that have been documented in both men and women. Men and women alike are vulnerable to "jet lag," "Monday morning blues" and *seasonal affective disorder*, a type of depression linked to the yearly change of seasons (and daylight hours). And both men and women show mood changes linked to infertility, even if it is their partner who has been diagnosed.

FICTION: Women with PMS are prone to violent outbursts and shouldn't be trusted.

FACT: Although crime rates, accidents, and suicide rates do appear to be higher among women during the two weeks preceding menstruation, *the rates for women are still much lower than the rates of violent acts committed by men.*

FICTION: If a remedy for PMS is written up in a scientific journal, it must work.

FACT: Our society tends to hold scientists in awe and to believe "scientific evidence" without questioning the way the results were obtained and whether they are scientifically valid. After all, you say, that's the job of the scientists. But just as some magazines and newspapers are more reputable than others, so it is with scientific journals, the studies published in them, and the scientists who carry out the research. Indeed, while hundreds of studies on PMS and various treatments have been published over the years, many of the earlier studies are now considered flawed and the conclusions in those studies have been called into question. One reason has to do with what is known as the *placebo response*, a phenomenon in which a patient's anticipation that a particular treatment will work is so high that even a sugar pill relieves symptoms. Among women with PMS, the placebo response is estimated to be about 50 percent. But placebo responses of up to 84 percent have been reported among women taking oral medication. And at least one study has found an astounding 94 percent placebo response with surgically inserted hormone implants. In other words, the "fake" implant was found to be as effective in relieving symptoms as the hormone-containing one. For this reason, any reliable study reporting on a potential treatment for PMS must include a comparison (or control) group of women who take a placebo. What's more, the experiment should be set up so that while it is in progress, the volunteers and the physicians who deal with them are "blinded;" in other words, neither the researchers nor the study participants know which volunteers are taking the active drug and which are taking the placebo. The more rigorous studies are designed so that the women taking the placebo during the first half of the study "cross over," or are switched to the active drug during the second half of the study, and vice versa. This is what is known as a *double-blind, placebo-controlled, crossover study*. Finally, the study should be carried out for at least three months—long enough for any placebo response to wear off and for the true effectiveness of the treatment to become apparent. So when we discuss an effective treatment in this book, we mean one that has been scientifically proven in a double-blind, placebo-controlled, crossover study. If a therapeutic regimen discussed in this book has not met this rigorous scientific criteria, we'll tell you. You should look for the same scientific evidence in the news reports of new "treatment breakthroughs" for PMS—even those appearing in the scientific journals. If the study isn't at least placebo-controlled, you should be skeptical of the results. Keep in mind, too, that even the advice in this book is subject to change as new and better scientific findings take the place of old ones. So be flexible and try to keep up with the medical advances as much as you can. And *always* double-check the source of the information, which often is as important as the information itself; the most reliable sources are double-blind, placebo-controlled, crossover studies.

FICTION: There's no treatment for PMS, so I'll just have to learn to live with it.

FACT: This is perhaps the biggest myth of all. While there's no cure for PMS, a majority of women respond well to a combination of counseling, life-style changes and, when necessary, medications for specific symptoms. Women with severe PMS may benefit from what we call "syndromal therapy" in which a woman's reproductive hormonal pattern is altered, providing treatment for the entire syndrome, not just specific symptoms. What's more, the most important member of your treatment team is you. In the pages that follow, you'll learn how to work with your physician to develop a treatment program that's right for you. But first, you should learn as much as you can about premenstrual syndrome, how it affects you, and its possible causes.

FINDING THE RIGHT PHYSICIAN

If you suspect you have PMS, you'll want to find a sympathetic doctor, preferably one who keeps abreast of the latest research and treatments associated with the condition. But which type of doctor should you see—a gynecologist or a mental health professional such as a psychiatrist?

The answer is probably both. More and more experts now see the wisdom of taking a team approach to treatment. The treatment team may include a gynecologist who is familiar with your reproductive and physical health and who can help with such physical symptoms as breast tenderness, as well as a psychologist or other mental health professional, who can help you learn coping strategies for dealing with emotional flare-ups. Some women may find a nutrition counselor or dietitian helpful, as well. (For help in locating one of these professionals, ask your regular doctor for a referral, or see our Recommended Resources, on page 144.)

This team approach is one advantage of going to one of the many PMS clinics that have sprung up around the country over the last ten years. Often, these clinics offer the services of many health professionals, such as a gynecologist, an internist (a physician who specializes in the treatment of "internal" organs, such as the heart and endocrine [hormonal] system), a psychiatrist or psychologist, and a nutritionist, all under one roof.

Sometimes, however, convenience has a price: some PMS clinics may recommend more—and more costly—diagnostic tests than you really need. Other clinics may tout unproven remedies, such as vitamin supplements. Of course, this is true of some physicians in private practice, as well, so let the buyer beware.

Your best protection against less-than-reputable physicians and clinics is knowledge—knowledge about how PMS is diagnosed, and about which treatment strategies have met the burden of scientific proof and which have not. So read on.

CHAPTER 2

WHAT IS PMS?

Children and teenage girls who are not yet menstruating don't have PMS. Pregnant and nursing women don't complain of premenstrual symptoms. Neither do most postmenopausal women or women in their childbearing years who, for one reason or another, aren't ovulating. The symptoms of PMS are inextricably linked to a woman's monthly menstrual cycle. But how?

Before we look at some of the many theories that have been proposed to explain PMS, you should have a basic understanding of your reproductive system and menstrual cycle.

YOUR REPRODUCTIVE SYSTEM AND MENSTRUAL CYCLE

Two key organs in your reproductive system are the *ovaries* (see Figure 1), which contain hundreds of thousands of immature eggs, each surrounded by a sac of cells known as a *primary follicle*. Every month during your reproductive years, a single egg, or *ovum*, ripens and is released from one of your ovaries, a process called *ovulation*.

Your uterus also plays a major role in the reproductive cycle. The uterus is a pear-shaped muscular cavity where a growing fetus receives nourishment and protection throughout pregnancy (see Figure 1). Each month, the uterine lining, or *endometrium*, thickens in preparation for pregnancy. If an egg

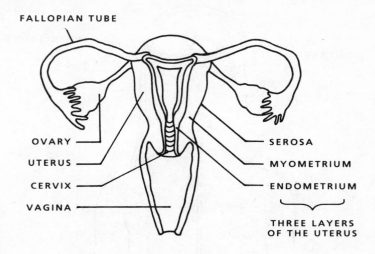

FALLOPIAN TUBE

OVARY

UTERUS

CERVIX

VAGINA

SEROSA

MYOMETRIUM

ENDOMETRIUM

THREE LAYERS
OF THE UTERUS

FIGURE 1 Female reproductive organs.

isn't fertilized and pregnancy doesn't occur, the endometrium is shed, a process known as *menstruation*.

Central to the operation of your reproductive organs are two specialized glands at the base of the brain: the hypothalamus and the pituitary gland (see Figure 2). The hypothalamus is one of the "master glands" in the body that controls the *endocrine (glandular) system*, a network of specialized organs (including the ovaries) that communicate with each other through the secretion of chemical messengers known as *hormones*. The hypothalamus regulates such basic bodily functions as water balance, body temperature, sleep, and food intake. This part of the brain is also instrumental in evoking strong emotional reactions, notably anger. In addition, the hypothalamus is responsible for the development of secondary sexual characteristics around the time of puberty, such as the growth of pubic hair, the development of breasts, and the accumulation of body fat around the buttocks and shoulders.

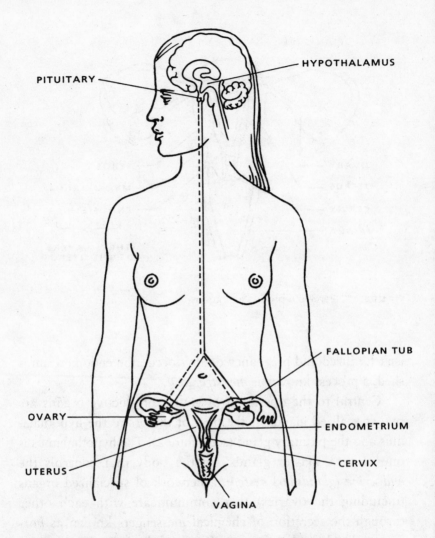

FIGURE 2 Female reproductive system. Your reproductive organs are governed by hormones secreted by the hypothalamus and pituitary glands. The hypothalamus secretes *gonadotropin releasing hormone* (GRH), which signals the pituitary gland to secrete *follicle stimulating hormone* (FSH) and *luteinizing hormone* (LH). These hormones stimulate an egg sac in one of the ovaries to grow. As the egg matures, the egg sac secretes the hormones *estrogen* and *progesterone*, which thicken the uterine lining in preparation for pregnancy. Rising levels of these hormones suppress the release of FSH and LH from the pituitary. When pregnancy doesn't occur, estrogen and progesterone levels fall off and the uterine lining is shed. The lower levels of estrogen and progesterone cause the pituitary gland to once again begin releasing FSH and LH, and the cycle begins again.

The pituitary gland is a small gland attached to and controlled by the hypothalamus. The pituitary gland consists of two portions: the anterior lobe and the posterior lobe. The anterior lobe is the more important one for purposes of our discussion. Hormones released from this part of the pituitary gland control other endocrine glands throughout the body, including the thyroid gland, the mammary (milk-producing) glands in the breasts, and the ovaries.

YOUR REPRODUCTIVE HORMONES

Your monthly menstrual cycle is governed by a complex interplay of hormones secreted by the hypothalamus, the pituitary gland, and the ovaries. The major reproductive hormones are:

Gonadotropin releasing hormone (GnRH)

This hormone, secreted by the hypothalamus, triggers the release of hormones from the pituitary gland.

Follicle stimulating hormone and luteinizing hormone

In response to GnRH from the hypothalamus, the pituitary gland secretes two hormones essential for the maturation and release of an egg from the ovaries. In the first few days after the start of your period, during what is known as the follicular phase of your menstrual cycle, the pituitary gland begins releasing *follicle stimulating hormone* (FSH), followed a few days later by *luteinizing hormone* (LH).

These hormones (see Figure 3), particularly FSH, stimulate the growth of six to twelve primary follicles in the ovaries. Eventually, the growth of one egg will begin to outpace the others, and only this egg will grow sufficiently to ripen and be released from one of your ovaries. The other follicles stop growing and begin to disintegrate.

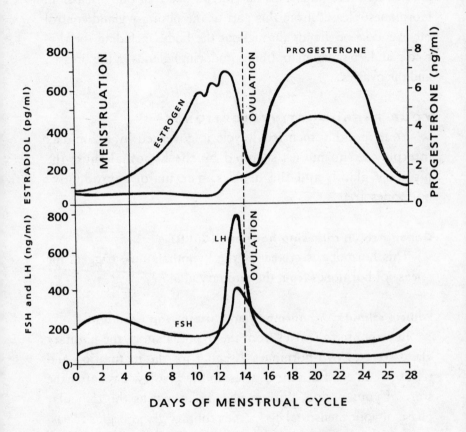

FIGURE 3 Levels of reproductive hormones throughout the menstrual cycle.

In the middle of your menstrual cycle—around day fourteen if you have a normal twenty-eight day cycle—the pituitary gland releases a surge of luteinizing hormone. This causes the growing follicle to swell rapidly and causes the wall of the follicle to weaken. Within hours, the follicle ruptures, releasing the ovum into the abdominal cavity. The tiny hairs at the opening of the fallopian tubes almost always draw the egg into the tube, where it can be fertilized.

Estrogen

As the follicles mature, they begin producing estrogen (see Figure 3). This hormone stimulates the cells lining your uterus to grow and thicken, helping to prepare the uterus for pregnancy.

Progesterone

After ovulation, the cells lining the ruptured follicle form what is known as the *corpus luteum*. This mass of yellow cells secretes small amounts of estrogen and large amounts of progesterone (see Figure 3), which further help thicken the uterine lining. This is known as the *luteal phase* of your menstrual cycle.

Rising levels of progesterone, together with estrogen and another hormone produced by the corpus luteum, known as *inhibin*, also signal the pituitary gland to stop producing FSH and LH.

The corpus luteum depends on FSH and LH to sustain it. So when FSH and LH levels fall, the corpus luteum begins to degenerate. This results in a sudden drop in estrogen and progesterone, which in turn, causes the endometrial lining to degenerate. A day or two later, the uterine lining is shed from the walls of the uterus, and you begin menstruating.

In the meantime, the pituitary gland, with no estrogen, progesterone, and inhibin to suppress it, begins secreting FSH and LH once again, stimulating more follicles and beginning the cycle anew. The whole process takes about twenty-eight days. But it's perfectly normal to have a menstrual cycle that lasts as few as twenty-one days or as many as thirty-five days.

WHAT CAUSES PMS?

Because PMS affects both mind and body, theories about its causes are almost as wide-ranging as the symptoms themselves. Research thus far has focused mostly on physiological causes, such as progesterone, endorphins in the brain, thyroid hormones, and the like. But as with most illnesses, there is probably more than one cause of PMS. Some of the major theories now being developed include the following:

ESTROGEN AND PROGESTERONE

These two hormones have long been suspected of somehow triggering the symptoms of PMS. One look at the association between premenstrual symptoms and fluctuating levels of estrogen and progesterone in menstruating women can tell you why (see Figure 4).

The idea that PMS was caused by a deficiency of the hormone progesterone was first put forth in the 1930s and 1940s, when it was believed that many of the symptoms of PMS were caused by excessive amounts of estrogen. Based on this theory, Katharina Dalton, M.D., a British gynecologist, began giving progesterone to women with PMS. According to her reports, the treatment relieved symptoms in almost all the women who took progesterone. Her 1977 book *The Premenstrual Syndrome and Progesterone Therapy* (reissued in 1984) popularized the use of progesterone suppositories to treat PMS.

Since that time, numerous studies have found no evidence whatsoever that women with PMS have lower levels of proges-

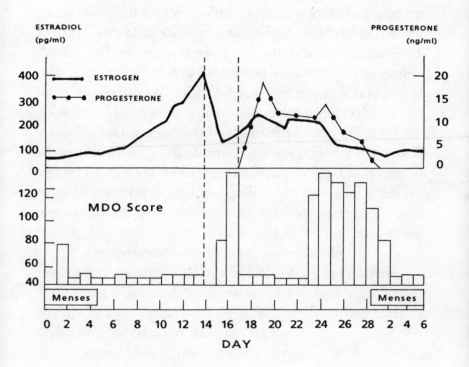

FIGURE 4 Hormonal changes and premenstrual symptoms. The top graph shows the fluctuations in levels of estrogen and progesterone over the course of the menstrual cycle; the bottom graph shows the rise and fall of premenstrual symptoms of depression and irritability during the same length of time, symptoms measured by the MDQ, Moos' Menstrual Distress Questionnaire. Notice how increased levels of PMS symptoms correspond with falling levels of the two hormones; for instance, the fall in estrogen on days 14 through 16 leads to increased symptoms on the same days, and the symptoms increase again on day 23 of the cycle, corresponding with the fall of both hormones.

terone than women who don't suffer premenstrual symptoms. Nor is there any scientific proof that women with PMS have either excesses or deficiencies of any other reproductive hormones, including estrogen, follicle stimulating hormone, luteinizing hormone, testosterone, or other androgens. Then in 1990 came a major study from Ellen Freeman, Ph.D., and colleagues at the University of Pennsylvania in Philadelphia, who found that progesterone suppositories overall are no more effective than a placebo in alleviating premenstrual symptoms.

There are other problems with the progesterone deficiency theory. For instance, Barbara Parry, M.D., a psychiatrist at the University of California at San Diego, points out that if a progesterone shortage were the culprit, women with PMS would experience more than their fair share of infertility. But this simply hasn't been the case, at least among the more than 600 patients who have sought treatment in Dr. Parry's PMS program.

Even among the handful of studies suggesting that women with PMS *do* have a progesterone deficiency, it's not clear whether the lower levels of progesterone are a cause of PMS or a consequence of it, since lack of sleep and other stressors associated with premenstrual syndrome itself could decrease progesterone levels.

In spite of these findings, a hormonal basis for PMS still can't be discounted altogether. It's possible that women with PMS may simply be more sensitive to relatively minor fluctuations in normal levels of hormones than other women. However, the current technology for measuring blood hormone levels is not yet sophisticated enough to test this theory.

In a 1989 scientific paper published in a British medical journal, Dr. Dalton suggests that women with PMS may have underactive progesterone receptors (specialized parts on the surface of cells that attract and bind the hormone to the cells), and that high levels of progesterone or certain levels of estrogen are needed to activate these receptors. Another possibility is that women with PMS experience progesterone-related withdrawal symptoms, since premenstrual symptoms typically worsen when progesterone levels fall just before menstruation.

ESTROGEN AND ENDORPHINS

Still other theories have focused on the effects of estrogen and progesterone on the brain. In rats, estrogen and progesterone have a direct effect on certain parts of the brain, particularly the hypothalamus. What's more, there's some evidence that estrogen affects the activity of natural pain-relieving chemicals known as *endorphins* in the hypothalamus. In rats and rhesus monkeys, removal of the estrogen-producing ovaries decreases the activity of endorphins, whereas estrogen replacement therapy increases endorphin activity. And endorphin activity appears to be influenced by the menstrual cycle itself; endorphin activity is highest during the middle part of the menstrual cycle's luteal phase, when estrogen and progesterone levels are elevated, and falls dramatically just before menstruation.

Endorphins are powerful—and highly addictive—substances. Synthetic narcotics, such as morphine, can produce a physical dependence in as little as seventy hours after you start taking them. So it's possible that the increased endorphin activity triggered by elevated estrogen and progesterone levels leads to a temporary addiction. And the abrupt withdrawal of endorphins just before menstruation may trigger withdrawal symptoms similar to those experienced by drug addicts. Indeed, irritability, anxiety, depression, increased appetite, vague abdominal cramps accompanied by loose bowel movements or actual diarrhea, insomnia and headaches—all symptoms frequently experienced by women in the days just before menstruation—are well-known signs of narcotics withdrawal.

ESTROGEN, PROGESTERONE, AND SEROTONIN

Also under investigation is whether or not estrogen and progesterone affect certain brain chemicals—notably *serotonin*. Serotonin is one of many *neurotransmitters* that help nerve cells in the brain and elsewhere in the body to communicate with one another. Low levels of serotonin have been associated with an increased incidence of depression, aggressive behavior, and social isolation—symptoms similar to those associated with PMS.

We (authors Rapkin and colleagues) found that blood serotonin levels were significantly lower during the last ten days of the menstrual cycle among women with PMS, while unaffected women experienced a rise in serotonin levels. In another study, we gave large doses of *tryptophan* (the amino acid building block of serotonin) to women with PMS and a comparison group of unaffected women at various times during the menstrual cycle. In the control women, the tryptophan consistently increased blood serotonin levels throughout all phases of the menstrual cycle. But women with PMS experienced a decrease in blood serotonin levels after taking tryptophan during the week before menstruation, pointing again to a premenstrual shortage of serotonin in women with PMS.

Rat studies suggest that estrogen and progesterone may influence the body's use and metabolism (breakdown) of serotonin, which could help explain why women with PMS have lower levels of serotonin after ovulation. But since all women experience the same hormonal fluctuations during the menstrual cycle, why wouldn't *all* women have low serotonin levels after ovulation and be susceptible to the same premenstrual symptoms? Apparently, serotonin levels are not governed by biology alone. Behavior—specifically social interaction—may influence serotonin levels in the body, as well. For instance, in the 1980s, sociobiologists Michael T. McGuire, M.D., and Michael J. Raleigh, Ph.D., at the University of California at Los Angeles, conducted a number of fascinating, well-designed studies on monkeys, and found that dominant males have blood serotonin levels significantly higher than those of nondominant males. But when dominant males are taken out of their social group and kept in isolation, serotonin levels fall within seven to ten days to the levels of nondominant males. And when nondominant males suddenly become dominant (after the dominant male has been removed from the group), they experience a marked increase in serotonin levels within seven to ten days.

Behavior and social interaction influence serotonin levels in humans, too. Higher levels of serotonin are found in "high status" men as opposed to "lower status" men. And men and women who engage in sensitive touching, such as hand-holding and stroking, also experience increased serotonin levels.

It's possible, then, that women without PMS seek out "serotonin fixes" in the form of rewarding social interactions—talking with an empathetic friend, for example—to help offset the lower serotonin levels triggered by ovulation. Women with PMS may not be as adept at getting these social "serotonin fixes," or may not be in a position to receive them. As a result, their social isolation could exacerbate the biological decline in serotonin triggered by ovulation, creating a downward spiral of lower serotonin levels, leading to increased social withdrawal, and even lower serotonin levels. If this is the case, it may be possible to develop a psychotherapy program to help women with PMS offset the biological decline in serotonin through positive behavioral changes.

ESTROGEN AND HEADACHES

Fluctuating estrogen levels throughout the menstrual cycle may also be responsible for migraine headaches that many women experience just before menstruation, what are often referred to as *menstrual migraines*. These are severe headaches usually accompanied by nausea, vomiting, and sensitivity to light or sound that typically occur in the week before or the week of menstruation. Women with menstrual migraines generally don't experience these severe headaches at other times during the menstrual cycle. If you are susceptible to migraine headaches at other times in the menstrual cycle, you probably *don't* have menstrual migraines. However, many migraine sufferers do notice a worsening of their headaches just before menstruation. It's important to distinguish between migraines and menstrual migraines, since each is treated differently.

Migraine headaches themselves are believed to be caused by constriction of blood vessels in the brain followed by dilation of the blood vessels. Menstrual migraines are believed to be triggered by a drop in estrogen after a period of several days' exposure to high estrogen levels. Falling estrogen levels are thought somehow to make the blood vessels in the brain more sensitive to other brain chemicals (possibly even serotonin) that cause the blood vessels to constrict, triggering a migraine. This theory helps explain why women with menstrual migraines experience worse symptoms when they take estrogen-containing oral contraceptives (which cause an even greater premenstrual drop in estrogen levels than the naturally-occurring fall in estrogen during the menstrual cycle), and why these women usually become headache-free during pregnancy, when estrogen levels remain high. (For more information on the treatment of menstrual migraines, see page 85.)

FLUID RETENTION

Because so many women with PMS complain of weight gain, bloating, and fluid retention, researchers have long suspected that PMS may be related to hormones and chemicals responsible for fluid balance in the body. These include *aldosterone*, a hormone released by the adrenal glands that causes the kidneys to retain sodium and water, *angiotensin*, a chemical in the blood that constricts blood vessels and stimulates the release of aldosterone from the adrenal glands, and *renin*, an enzyme released by the kidneys that converts biologically inactive angiotensin in the blood into an active form. But researchers have found no significant differences in levels of these substances among women with PMS and comparison groups of unaffected women. Moreover, no studies have conclusively shown that women with PMS actually do gain weight, or that weight gain could be attributed to fluid retention.

One possibility may be that fluids are somehow redistributed in the body during the premenstrual phase of the menstrual cycle. In women with PMS, sodium and water are known to accumulate in the breasts, hands, and feet, and estrogen and progesterone may be partly responsible. Although the exact mechanisms are poorly understood, estrogen affects the renin-angiotensin-aldosterone network of hormones, raising aldosterone levels and causing sodium and water retention. Estrogen also increases blood flow throughout the body, leading to dilation of blood vessels in estrogen-responsive tissues, such as the breasts. Progesterone has the opposite effect, causing the kidneys to excrete sodium. Some researchers suspect the body may compensate for this by releasing more aldosterone, ultimately resulting in increased fluid retention during the last half of the menstrual cycle.

Another possible cause of fluid retention among some women may be premenstrual cravings for sweets and salty foods. G. A. MacGregor, M.D., a British physician, in 1979 showed that women who switched from a normal diet to a low-sodium, low-carbohydrate diet, then to a high-sodium, high-carbohydrate diet experienced a weight gain of as much as ten pounds in twenty-four hours.

You should be aware, however, that no studies have conclusively been able to demonstrate an increased incidence or severity of depression, irritability, or other emotional symptoms associated with changes in body fluid.

PROLACTIN

This hormone, secreted by the pituitary gland, is involved in the development of the breasts and in breast milk production. Because of its direct effect on the breasts, prolactin has been suspected of causing the breast tenderness that many women experience just before their periods. Prolactin is also suspected of playing a role in premenstrual fluid retention. The hormone does help regulate fluid balance in other animals, and some women with apparent premenstrual fluid retention also have been found to have abnormally high levels of prolactin, a condition known as *hyperprolactinemia*. However, researchers at the National Institute of Mental Health and elsewhere have found that while prolactin levels do fluctuate throughout a woman's menstrual cycle, there are no significant differences in levels of prolactin between PMS sufferers and nonsufferers. Nor do all women with hyperprolactinemia experience premenstrual symptoms. Nevertheless, one drug that suppresses prolactin secretion (*bromocriptine*, brand name Parlodel) is effective in relieving the breast tenderness associated with PMS, although it doesn't improve other premenstrual symptoms.

PROSTAGLANDINS

These substances, produced in such tissues as the brain, breasts, blood vessels, gastrointestinal tract, kidney, and reproductive tract, are thought to play an important role in the regulation of many different bodily functions by interacting with other prostaglandins and hormones. For this reason, researchers theorize that prostaglandin imbalances could possibly influence symptoms associated with PMS. Levels of the breast-milk producing hormone prolactin, for instance, are influenced by prostaglandins that cause dilation of the blood vessels and breast tenderness. Prostaglandins produced in the central nervous system—notably a prostaglandin known as PGE1—act like neurotransmitters to modify thirst, appetite, temperature, mood, and certain hormones. Some researchers think these prostaglandins may produce symptoms typical of PMS, such as headache, fatigue, and cravings for sweets.

In the kidneys, blood flow and fluid balances are tied to prostaglandin actions, which could theoretically lead to the fluid retention associated with PMS. And prostaglandins produced in the uterine lining are believed to be responsible for premenstrual cramping, diarrhea, and nausea. Indeed, changes in prostaglandin levels have been associated with several problems linked to the reproductive system, notably *dysmenorrhea* ("painful periods"), *menorrhagia* (heavy periods), and *endometriosis*, a condition in which the lining of the uterus grows outside of the uterine cavity. Interestingly, women with dysmenorrhea appear to be somewhat prone to PMS and vice versa. And PMS is frequently associated with endometriosis. Still, there's no concrete evidence that prostaglandin imbalances are responsible for premenstrual symptoms.

HYPOGLYCEMIA

Many women with PMS complain of food cravings and increased appetite, along with fatigue, dizziness, headaches, shakiness, and cold sweats. Because these symptoms are similar to those associated with low blood sugar, or *hypoglycemia*, some researchers began to suspect that women with PMS may actually be suffering from episodes of hypoglycemia. So far, there's no evidence that women with PMS have blood sugar levels lower than 50 mg/dL during the time the women report having "hypoglycemic attacks." However, some studies have shown that women with PMS do have greater swings in blood sugar levels during the latter half of the menstrual cycle, which could account for premenstrual symptoms of hypoglycemia. Skipping meals and cutting back on food to offset the bloating associated with PMS may make the problem even worse by keeping blood sugar levels low.

NUTRITIONAL DEFICIENCIES

Because women with PMS experience food cravings, a number of researchers have suggested that nutritional deficiencies may influence premenstrual symptoms. A possible deficiency in vitamin B_6 has received the most attention. The connection between vitamin B_6 and the menstrual cycle was first made back in the 1940s, when it was thought that excessive estrogen levels (resulting from a deficiency in progesterone) might interfere with the liver's metabolism of B vitamins, causing a vitamin deficiency. The theory was fueled by poorly designed studies showing that vitamin B_6 supplements relieved premenstrual symptoms. Then came reports that women with severe vitamin B_6 deficiencies had normal levels of estrogen, which discredited the theory.

Vitamin B_6 has received renewed interest because of its role in the manufacture of the brain chemicals dopamine and serotonin. As mentioned earlier, a deficiency of these neurotransmitters has been implicated as a cause of naturally occurring depression. Lower dopamine levels also result in an excess of the hormone aldosterone in the body, which may lead to salt and fluid retention. So a deficiency in dopamine or serotonin might explain the PMS symptoms of anxiety, irritability, depression, and fluid retention. Vitamin B_6 increases dopamine and serotonin levels and has a sedative effect. But no studies have found either an outright or minor vitamin B_6 deficiency among women with PMS.

Another nutrient receiving increased scrutiny for a possible role in PMS is magnesium. Researchers have found lower blood levels of magnesium in women with PMS, particularly those who crave sweets. And a 1991 study by Fabio Facchinetti, M.D., and colleagues at the University of Pavia in Italy has shown that magnesium supplements may help ease some PMS symptoms. No one is certain how magnesium works. A magnesium deficiency may cause lower levels of the neurotransmitter dopamine, which could trigger depression.

PSYCHOLOGICAL DISORDERS

Premenstrual syndrome and major depression share many of the same symptoms, such as feelings of hopelessness, blue moods, a decreased interest in things, fatigue, sleep disturbances, and appetite changes. Because of these similarities, researchers have begun investigating a possible link between premenstrual syndrome and other emotional disorders, particularly major clinical depression. Depression in women has already been associated with other times in a woman's reproductive life, including *menarche* (the start of menstruation), the use of oral contraceptives, pregnancy, infertility, miscarriage through the twentieth week of pregnancy, or loss of a fetus after the twentieth week, which is even more traumatic, and menopause. In one study, about 30 percent of women with recurring depression experienced their first depressive episode during a period of reproductive hormonal change, such as after pregnancy.

From 50 to 75 percent of women who have been diagnosed with depression experience premenstrual depression. And there's evidence that a woman who has premenstrual depression is more likely to experience a major depressive episode at some point in her life. Moreover, symptoms associated with such psychological disorders as anxiety and depression are known to worsen during the latter half of the menstrual cycle among affected women. Some researchers estimate that up to 50 percent of women who seek medical help for PMS actually suffer from underlying anxiety or depression.

CIRCADIAN RHYTHMS

New research suggests that abnormalities in the body's circadian rhythms, or "biological clock," may contribute to the premenstrual depression some women experience. Desynchronization of the body's biological clock, the internal timing mechanism that regulates such functions as sleep, body temperature fluctuations, and hormonal secretions, is already suspected of causing seasonal depression and other cyclic disorders.

One marker of the body's biological clock is the hormone *melatonin*, which is secreted only at night by the pineal gland in the brain. In a 1990 study, Barbara Parry, M.D., and colleagues at the University of California at San Diego found that eight women with PMS had significantly lower blood levels of melatonin during the luteal phase of the menstrual cycle than eight unaffected women. Low levels of melatonin, a derivative of serotonin, have also been found in people suffering from depression and could be responsible for the mood swings associated with premenstrual syndrome.

A handful of small studies also shows that therapy involving exposure to bright lights or forced sleep extension or deprivation can help reset the body's biological clock, possibly helping to relieve symptoms of PMS in some women.

Even after more than fifty years of research, scientists still don't have a good understanding of what causes PMS, which can be a real source of frustration for you. You can take comfort in knowing that our knowledge of PMS is increasing every day. So are the ways in which women like you can be helped. But before we look at some of the treatments for PMS, we will first discuss how a diagnosis is made.

CHAPTER 3

DO YOU HAVE PMS?

Although it may take a month or two for your doctor to make a formal diagnosis of PMS, it is essential to ensure that you receive proper treatment. An incorrect diagnosis can lead to years of ineffective therapy—and needless suffering on your part. Since no reliable laboratory tests have yet been developed to diagnose PMS, and since symptoms may mimic those associated with other physical or psychological problems, your physician will generally begin by ruling out other possible causes of the symptoms. Here's a look at what you can expect.

THE PHYSICAL EXAMINATION AND MEDICAL HISTORY

A physical examination can help uncover other medical conditions that may cause symptoms similar to PMS, such as thyroid problems, diabetes, or over-activity of the adrenal glands. Depending on your symptoms, this examination may include the following:

MEDICAL HISTORY

A thorough medical history can help your physician ferret out past or current medical conditions that could be causing or exacerbating your symptoms. Be sure to make a note of the date of your last menstrual period before your appointment.

You'll be asked. It's also a good idea to make a list of all your symptoms—even those that don't appear to be cyclical. Better yet, start keeping a record of your symptoms now so that when you see your doctor, you'll be able to tell him or her whether your symptoms correspond with your menstrual cycle. (Use the PMS Diary on pages 47–51.) Be sure to be up front about your use of alcohol and drugs, too. Sometimes symptoms of a chemical dependency mimic those of PMS.

PHYSICAL EXAMINATION

The examination will likely include a routine blood pressure check, a pelvic exam and Pap smear, a breast examination by your physician, and other routine tests.

BLOOD TESTS

These may include a complete blood count and chemistry screen to rule out anemia and other chronic illness, such as kidney or liver problems (these are rare). If your symptoms include fatigue and irritability, your physician may recommend that you undergo a *thyroid function test* to determine whether you have a thyroid disorder. All of these tests require only that you have blood drawn from your arm. If you have high blood pressure (hypertension) or diabetes and complain of depression, your doctor may order blood tests for *Cushing's syndrome*, a disorder caused by over-production of cortisol by the adrenal glands or from the use of certain drugs.

You should be aware that expensive hormone tests used by some PMS clinics in the initial evaluation are usually not necessary to make a diagnosis. Remember: researchers have found no demonstrable changes in blood hormone levels among women with PMS. However, if you are close to menopause and have some symptoms of menopause (including hot flashes), your physician may recommend that you undergo a blood test for levels of *follicle stimulating hormone* (FSH). High levels of FSH indicate that your ovaries' production of estrogen is down and that your symptoms may actually be early signs of menopause.

THE SYMPTOMS CHART

Once a physician has ruled out other possible causes of your symptoms, charting your symptoms *for at least two months* is the only definitive way to diagnose PMS. Why so long? To begin with, your symptoms may vary widely from cycle to cycle in both their timing and intensity, so you will need to record your symptoms for more than one menstrual cycle before a pattern begins to emerge. Keeping a record also helps you and your physician pinpoint your most bothersome symptoms, which can be used to help develop a treatment plan tailored to your needs.

There are two other good reasons to chart your symptoms: many women find that keeping track of their symptoms is therapeutic in itself. Moreover, charting your symptoms after you've begun treatment is the best way to determine whether the treatment is working.

PMS DIARY

Using the PRISM Calendar here, rate your symptoms every day, beginning on the first day of your menstrual cycle (the first day of your period). (If you don't want to wait until the start of your next menstrual period to begin charting your symptoms, count the number of days since the start of your last menstrual period and begin charting your symptoms from that day in your cycle.)

Don't try to rely on your recollections of past menstrual cycles to make a diagnosis. Studies have shown that doing so may lead to an inaccurate diagnosis. To make remembering easier, keep your

PRISM Calendar and a pen or pencil at your bedside and chart your symptoms just before you go to sleep at night, when the day's events and your symptoms are still fresh in your mind.

PRISM CALENDAR

Instructions for completing this calendar

1) On the first day of menstruation, prepare the calendar. Consider the first day of bleeding as day 1 of your menstrual cycle and enter the corresponding calendar date for each day in the space provided.

2) Each morning: Weigh yourself on the same scale after emptying your bladder and before eating breakfast. Record your baseline weight at the top of the chart, and any weight change from baseline in the space provided on the calendar.

3) Each evening: At about the same time, complete the column for that day as follows:

> **BLEEDING:** Indicate if you have had bleeding by shading the box above that day's date ■ ; for spotting, use an ⊠
>
> **SYMPTOMS:** If you experience symptoms, indicate their severity using the following scale:
>
> > Mild: **1** (noticeable but not troublesome)
> > Moderate: **2** (interferes with normal activity)
> > Severe: **3** (temporarily incapacitating)
>
> **LIFESTYLE IMPACT:** If the listed phrase applies to you that day, enter an ⊠
>
> **LIFE EVENTS:** If you experience one of the following events on that day, enter an ⊠
>
> > **Experiences:** For positive (happy) or negative (sad or disappointing) experiences unrelated to your symptoms, specify the nature of the events on the reverse side of this form.
> >
> > **Social Activities:** These include events, such as a special dinner, show, or party, involving family or friends.
> >
> > **Vigorous Exercise:** Participating in a sporting event or exercise program lasting more than 30 minutes.
>
> **MEDICATION:** In the bottom three rows, list medications if any and indicate days when taken by entering an ⊠.

The Prospective Record of the Impact and Severity of Menstrual Symptomatology (PRISM Calendar) reprinted from Reid, R. L., "Premenstrual Syndrome," in Current Problems in Obstetrics, Gynecology and Fertility, Vol. 8., No. 1, (1985), pages 5–57, with permission from Mosby-Year Book, Inc.

Baseline weight on day 1: _____ lbs

BLEEDING

Day of Menstrual Cycle	1	2	3	4	5	6	7	8	9	10	11	12	13	14	15	16	17	18	19	20	21	22	23	24	25	26	27	28	29	30	31	32	33	34	35	36	37	38	39	40
Month Date																																								
WEIGHT CHANGE																																								

SYMPTOMS

	1	2	3	4	5	6	7	8	9	10	11	12	13	14	15	16	17	18	19	20	21	22	23	24	25	26	27	28	29	30	31	32	33	34	35	36	37	38	39	40
Irritable																																								
Fatigue																																								
Inward anger																																								
Labile mood (crying)																																								
Depressed																																								
Restless																																								
Anxious																																								
Insomnia																																								
Lack of control																																								
Edema (swelling) or rings tight																																								
Breast tenderness																																								

Day of Menstrual Cycle	1	2	3	4	5	6	7	8	9	10	11	12	13	14	15	16	17	18	19	20	21	22	23	24	25	26	27	28	29	30	31	32	33	34	35	36	37	38	39	40
Month Date																																								

SYMPTOMS

Constipation																																								
Loose bowels																																								
Appetite ↑ up; ↓ down																																								
Chills (C); Sweats (S)																																								
Headaches																																								
Sweet cravings																																								
Salt cravings																																								
Feel unattractive																																								
Guilty																																								
Unreasonable behavior																																								
Low self-image																																								
Nausea																																								
Menstrual cramps																																								

Day of Menstrual Cycle	1	2	3	4	5	6	7	8	9	10	11	12	13	14	15	16	17	18	19	20	21	22	23	24	25	26	27	28	29	30	31	32	33	34	35	36	37	38	39	40
Month Date																																								

LIFESTYLE IMPACT

Physically aggressive																																								
Verbally aggressive																																								
Wish to be alone																																								
Neglect housework																																								
Time off work																																								
Disorganized/distractable																																								
Accident prone/clumsy																																								
Uneasy about driving																																								
Suicidal thoughts																																								
Stayed at home																																								
Increased use of alcohol																																								

Day of Menstrual Cycle	1	2	3	4	5	6	7	8	9	10	11	12	13	14	15	16	17	18	19	20	21	22	23	24	25	26	27	28	29	30	31	32	33	34	35	36	37	38	39	40
Month Date																																								

LIFE EVENTS

Negative experience																																								
Positive experience																																								
Social activities																																								
Vigorous exercise																																								

MEDICATIONS

BASAL BODY TEMPERATURE CHART

Charting your time of ovulation goes hand-in-hand with charting your symptoms. With a record of your monthly releases of an egg, you and your physician can determine whether your symptoms truly are premenstrual. This is especially important if you don't have regular menstrual cycles (women approaching menopause often don't). The best way to determine your time of ovulation is to take your basal body temperature (your body's resting temperature) every morning before you get out of bed. You'll need to use a special basal thermometer with large, easy-to-read temperature increments (most drugstores carry these) and the basal temperature chart here.

To determine your time of ovulation using your basal temperature:

1) Start taking your temperature on the first day of your menstrual cycle (the day your period begins), noting the month and date in the chart provided for you here. Mark the dates of your period with an *x* (see Figure 5).

2) Shake down the thermometer to 96 degrees Fahrenheit (35 degrees Celsius) before taking your temperature. (Do this at night before you go to bed so the thermometer will be ready for use when you wake up in the morning.)

3) Take your temperature before getting out of bed in the morning. You can take your temperature either orally or rectally; just be sure to use the same method every time. Leave the thermometer in for a minimum of three minutes.

4) Record and plot your temperature in the chart here. Your temperature may drop slightly, then increase 0.4 to 1 degrees Fahrenheit *after* you have ovulated and will remain at this higher level until a day or two prior to your next menstrual period.

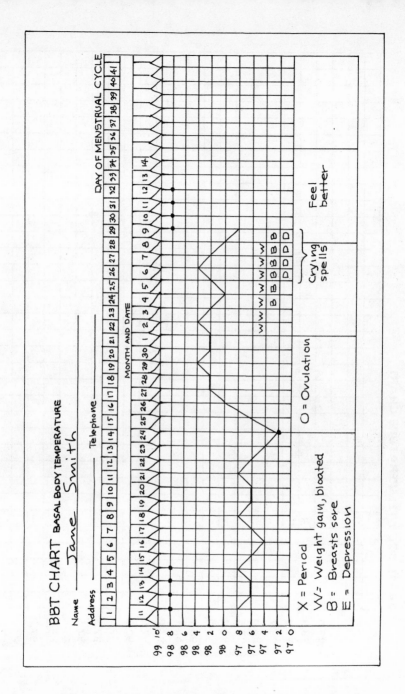

FIGURE 5 Sample basal body temperature chart. You will know that you have ovulated when your body temperature falls, rises slightly, and stays elevated, as shown in the chart here.

BASAL BODY TEMPERATURE CHART

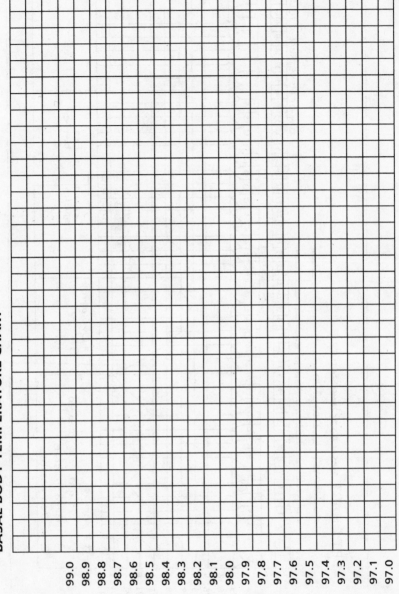

Month
Date
Day of Cycle
Temperature

99.0
98.9
98.8
98.7
98.6
98.5
98.4
98.3
98.2
98.1
98.0
97.9
97.8
97.7
97.6
97.5
97.4
97.3
97.2
97.1
97.0

FIGURE 5A Blank basal body temperature chart.

THE PSYCHOLOGICAL EVALUATION

If charting of your symptoms reveals that you have some symptoms—particularly depression, mood swings, anxiety, or other emotional symptoms—during the entire menstrual cycle, your physician may recommend that you undergo a psychological evaluation. Many women with emotional problems, such as depression or anxiety, experience a worsening of their symptoms prior to menstruation that may be mistaken for PMS. By some estimates, up to 50 percent of women seeking assistance for PMS actually suffer from underlying anxiety or depression, conditions that are best helped by proper medication and counseling.

Your physician may refer you to a qualified mental health professional for a psychological evaluation. The evaluation itself often consists of a standardized diagnostic interview. Or you may simply be asked to fill out one or more standardized questionnaires. When you have PMS, you will probably be asked to undergo a psychological evaluation both the week before and the week after your period to see if your menstrual cycle has any effect on the results. Women with PMS tend to have significantly lower mood scores on tests administered premenstrually.

IF YOU HAVE PMS . . .

You doctor will diagnose PMS if you meet the following criteria:

1) Your symptoms occur cyclically and recur to some degree in the luteal phase of your menstrual cycle (after ovulation).

2) During the follicular phase of your menstrual cycle (prior to ovulation), you are free of symptoms. You should experience at least seven symptom-free days in each cycle. (Some women

may experience symptoms near the time of ovulation that go away, then return during the week before menstruation.)

3) Your symptoms are severe enough to significantly alter your life-style (for instance, you regularly miss out on work during the days just preceding your period, or you have more fights with your spouse).

Even if you don't fulfill all of the above criteria, you may benefit from some of the self-care approaches described in the following two chapters. If you have severe PMS, these measures probably won't be enough to alleviate your symptoms, but one or more of the medications we discuss in Chapter 6 usually *will* make a difference.

CHAPTER 4

NUTRITIONAL THERAPIES: WORTH THEIR SALT?

Some of the most curious and bothersome symptoms associated with PMS are food cravings—particularly for carbohydrates, such as sweets, rolls, pasta, potatoes, and the like. For this reason, scientists have long questioned whether women with PMS suffered some kind of nutritional deficiency or processed food in a different way. And if a nutritional problem were responsible for some (or all) of a woman's premenstrual symptoms, the next logical step would be to correct the problem with some kind of nutritional therapy. Indeed, nutritional approaches to "female complaints" date back to the late nineteenth century, when the treatment of choice consisted of drinking a concoction of vegetable compounds dissolved in a watery solution containing 15 percent alcohol. In the 1930s, when "excessive estrogen" was blamed for causing premenstrual symptoms, women were advised to drink the laxative magnesium citrate to eliminate estrogen, along with plenty of coffee and tea, whose diuretic properties would presumably flush estrogen out through the kidneys. Calcium supplements were recommended as a sedative. In the 1940s, when PMS was thought to be caused by a vitamin B deficiency, rice bran and brewer's yeast were popular remedies. And in the 1950s, women were advised to cut back on carbohydrates and salt, and increase protein, mainly from dairy products, after female prisoners with PMS were observed to behave and perform better when these changes were made in their diets.

Even more recently, nutritional approaches to managing PMS are extremely popular. In a 1984 survey of 502 American physicians, 90 percent said they provided their patients with nutritional supplements for the management of PMS, and 60 percent said they recommended that their patients make dietary changes as well. Nutritional therapies are popular with women who suffer from PMS, too, because they're as close as your refrigerator door, they don't require a doctor's prescription, and most are safe and nutritionally sound. But you should be aware that most recommendations lack proof, and some—particularly those involving the use of megadoses of vitamins and minerals—may not be as harmless as they seem.

Here's a look at the facts behind some of the most common nutritional therapies for PMS so you can decide for yourself whether they're worth your time and trouble.

FOOD CRAVINGS: THE SEARCH FOR A CAUSE

A number of theories have been developed to explain why women with PMS experience increased appetite, food cravings, and other nutrition-related symptoms. Since many of the popular dietary recommendations for PMS are based on these theories, it pays to take a closer look at them.

NUTRITIONAL DEFICIENCIES

Some nutritional surveys have found that women with PMS consume three times more refined sugars as unaffected women, as well as more meat and dairy products, more caffeine and less B vitamins, iron, zinc, and magnesium. Some researchers, pointing to these survey results, have suggested that women with PMS suffer from nutritional deficiencies that lead to premenstrual symptoms, particularly shortages of vitamin B_6 and magnesium. So far, no studies have found evidence of outright deficiencies in Vitamin B_6, vitamin E, and most other nutrients among women with PMS. The only exception: magnesium. (You'll find more on these vitamins and minerals later in this chapter.) Still, measuring blood levels of vitamins and minerals doesn't always reveal a nutritional shortage within individual cells, and the technology for detecting vitamin and mineral deficiencies at the cellular level is still in its infancy.

Another problem is that it's impossible to tell from these surveys whether the women's poor eating habits caused their symptoms or their premenstrual food cravings drove them to make poor food choices.

LOW BLOOD SUGAR

As mentioned in Chapter 2, some premenstrual symptoms are similar to those associated with *hypoglycemia*, or abnormally low levels of glucose (a simple sugar) in the bloodstream. Hypoglycemia causes shakiness, sweating, dizziness, headache, irritability, anxiety, and fatigue. For this reason, some researchers have speculated that some premenstrual symptoms may actually be symptoms of hypoglycemia. Still, as we pointed out earlier, there's no evidence that women with PMS have blood sugar levels lower than 50 mg/dL during the time the women report having hypoglycemic attacks.

SEROTONIN SHORTAGES

Some of the more promising studies have suggested that carbohydrate cravings may be the body's way of compensating for low levels of serotonin in the brain, which are associated with depression. In 1988, Birgitta Both-Orthman, David Rubinow, M.D., and colleagues at the National Institute of Mental Health (NIMH) found that while all women experience an increased appetite during the last half of the menstrual cycle, women with PMS experience a much more dramatic increase in appetite than unaffected women. Moreover, the researchers found a significant relationship between the appetite of PMS sufferers and their mood in the premenstrual phase of their menstrual cycles only—as feelings of depression increased premenstrually, so did the women's hunger.

Similar findings have come from studies by Judith Wurtman, Ph.D., and colleagues at the Massachusetts Institute of Technology (MIT) in Cambridge. In one study, nineteen women with PMS and a comparison group of nine unaffected women actually lived in the MIT research center for two days during the premenstrual phase of their menstrual cycles and two days during the week just following menstruation. This gave the researchers much more control over the women's diets and a first-hand glimpse at their eating patterns. During their stay, the women were told to come to the dining room for meals, but they could eat as much or as little as they liked of three high-carbohydrate and three high-protein foods. In addition, the women had continuous access to six snacks stored in a refrigerated vending machine, such as cookies, candy, cheese, and cold cuts. The researchers found that women with PMS consumed significantly more food during the last half of the menstrual cycle than unaffected women, particularly carbohydrate-rich foods, including sweets *and* starchy carbohydrates, such as potatoes, bread, pasta, and rolls.

It's still not clear why women with PMS eat more foods, and more carbohydrate-rich foods just before their periods. Dr. Rubinow's group at the National Institute of Mental Health suggests that estrogen may work to suppress appetite in some way or that progesterone may somehow stimulate a woman's appetite. One possible mechanism of action: estrogen lowers dopamine levels, which in turn decreases brain levels of nore-pinephrine, a neurotransmitter believed to stimulate appetite.

A more likely explanation is that the major mood changes associated with PMS contribute to the large premenstrual increase in the appetites of affected women, just as a depressed mood appears to increase the appetite of women suffering from a type of depression known as *atypical depression*. People with seasonal affective disorder are also known to experience carbohydrate cravings in the autumn and winter, when seasonal depression sets in. The NIMH researchers suggest that the carbohydrate cravings of PMS, atypical depression, and seasonal affective disorder may be the body's way of compensating for low serotonin levels in the brain. Carbohydrates provide the tryptophan necessary to raise brain serotonin levels.

An experiment from Dr. Wurtman's laboratory adds weight to this theory. In a study related to the one mentioned earlier, eighteen women with PMS and fourteen unaffected women came to Dr. Wurtman's clinical research center once during the early follicular phase of their menstrual cycles and once during the late luteal phase. The women were instructed not to eat or drink anything after 3:00 P.M. on the day of their visit. When they arrived at the center, the women filled out three standardized questionnaires used to measure mood and sleepiness. Then the volunteers ate a "test meal" consisting of a high-carbohydrate bowl of corn flakes with a synthetic low-protein milk. An hour after eating the test meal, the women again filled out the same three questionnaires.

Women with PMS reported feeling significantly less depressed, tense, angry, confused, and tired and much more calm and alert after eating the high-carbohydrate test meal. The unaffected women reported no mood changes. What's more, the affected women's scores improved only during the few days just before the onset of menstruation. No mood changes were found among either group of women during the follicular test period. The researchers concluded that "individuals suffering from PMS may eat carbohydrates for their antidepressant effects."

This was not a placebo-controlled study and the study sample was small, so it's still too early to make sweeping dietary recommendations based on these findings. However, the research does provide a plausible explanation for carbohydrate food cravings among women with PMS.

BUT DO NUTRITIONAL THERAPIES WORK?

The burning question in the minds of most women with PMS (and the doctors who treat them) is whether or not you can manipulate your diet to ease food cravings and other premenstrual symptoms. Over the years, numerous dietary recommendations have been proposed to help relieve premenstrual symptoms. The most popular today include:

- Eat regular small meals
- Decrease your intake of salt, fat, sugar, and caffeine
- Increase your consumption of foods made from whole grains, legumes, seeds and nuts, vegetables, fruits, and vegetable oils.

You may also have heard that you should either increase or decrease your consumption of high-protein foods, such as meat and dairy products. Many women are told to take vitamin and mineral supplements, as well.

Since so much confusion surrounds these recommendations, let's look at how each one of them evolved, and whether or not there's enough evidence to substantiate the recommendations.

SMALL, FREQUENT MEALS

The recommendation to eat frequent, small meals arises from the still unproven theory that women with PMS experience episodes of hypoglycemia, or low blood sugar. Theoretically, eating three scaled down meals and plenty of wholesome between-meal snacks helps keep blood sugar levels on a more even keel, preventing the hypoglycemic episodes believed to trigger certain premenstrual symptoms.

Although no studies have documented improvements in premenstrual symptoms among women who follow this recommendation, many women do report that they feel better when they eat small, frequent meals. Since women with PMS do experience a sharply increased appetite during the second half of the menstrual cycle, eating regularly throughout the day could theoretically help take the edge off your hunger and may also help curb eating binges and food cravings. But again, there's no good, solid evidence that doing so will reduce these symptoms.

There may be other health benefits to this type of eating pattern, though. Some studies suggest that nibbling on small meals and healthful snacks throughout the day rather than gorging on three (or fewer) large meals may lower blood cholesterol levels (and hence reduce your risk of heart disease later in life).

This recommendation certainly can't hurt, and who knows . . . it just may help you feel better.

SODIUM

Your body uses sodium (the main component of table salt) to maintain its balance of fluids and electrolytes, and a diet high in sodium can cause you to retain water. So you can see why so many women with PMS are advised to cut back on sodium. In fact, reducing your sodium intake is perhaps the safest, most effective way to handle fluid retention associated with PMS. (As you'll see in Chapter 6, cutting back on sodium is often just as effective as over-the-counter diuretics and a whole lot safer.)

If fluid retention is one of your major symptoms, by all means, try reducing your sodium intake. Just remember that no research has found a connection between fluid retention and the psychological symptoms of PMS, such as irritability and depression. Nor has the research documented a premenstrual weight gain that could be directly attributed to edema. So don't expect to feel better emotionally or necessarily register a weight loss on the scale by cutting back on salt. You may, however, feel less bloated, notice less swelling, and feel physically more comfortable by reducing your salt intake in the week or two just before your period.

HOW TO CUT BACK ON SODIUM

The National Research Council says you can get by on as little as 500 mg of sodium per day. A more comfortable goal to aim for is between 1800 and 2400 mg per day, which is still far less than the 4,000 to 7,000 mg consumed by the average American. Here are some suggestions for shaking the salt habit:

- Cook your own foods. You have much more control over the sodium content of foods you prepare yourself. And while many foods naturally contain sodium, about a third of the average American's sodium intake comes from salt used in cooking and from the salt shaker on the table.
- Use spices, herbs, and other seasonings or a salt substitute instead of salt in cooking. Avoid vegetable

salts and flakes, such as onion, garlic, or celery salt, and celery or parsley flakes, which are high in sodium. Beware of products claiming to be "low sodium" salt substitutes. Most contain another salt *and* sodium chloride, and contain about half as much sodium (1100 mg per teaspoon) as regular table salt (2300 mg per teaspoon). That's still quite a lot of sodium. These are not salt substitutes.

- Substitute baking powder and baking soda with low-sodium leavening agents, such as cream of tartar, sodium-free baking powder, potassium bicarbonate, and yeast.

- Avoid prepackaged, processed, and fast foods (such as canned or frozen foods). These are notoriously high in sodium. Some foods to avoid include prepackaged frozen foods, frozen fish fillets and shellfish, frozen peas and lima beans, packaged mixes for sauces, gravies, casseroles and noodle, rice or potato dishes, canned soups, and all canned meat and vegetable products unless they have been prepared without salt.

- Beware of baked goods, such as breads, desserts, cakes, cookies, and quick-cooking or instant breakfast cereals, which contribute almost 30 percent of the sodium in the average diet. Better low-sodium choices include shredded wheat, puffed wheat or puffed rice, farina, grits, or oatmeal that you prepare yourself, and breads and rolls made without salt.

- Avoid smoked, processed, or cured meats and fish, such as ham, bacon, corned beef, cold cuts, frankfurters, sausage, tongue, salt pork, chipped beef, pickled herring, and anchovies. These are loaded with sodium.

- Avoid high-sodium meat extracts, bouillon cubes and meat sauces.
- Avoid salted snack foods, such as potato chips, crackers, nuts, and popcorn. Better snack choices are fresh fruits and raw vegetables. Fresh fruits and vegetables are naturally low in sodium, fat, and calories and high in vitamins and fiber, making them all around good, nutritious choices. If you must indulge in processed snack foods, buy unsalted chips and nuts and low-sodium crackers. Season your own (air popped) popcorn with a salt substitute or herbal seasoning blend.
- Go easy on prepared condiments, relishes, Worcestershire sauce, catsup, pickles, mustard, olives, soy sauce, and monosodium glutamate.
- Buy unsalted butter and peanut butter and low-sodium or no-salt-added cheeses.

SUGAR

Proponents of reducing sugar in your diet point out that simple sugars are more rapidly absorbed into your bloodstream and raise your blood sugar levels faster than most other foods. They speculate that the subsequent sharp rise in insulin (a hormone secreted by the pancreas that helps clear sugar from the bloodstream) could lead to hypoglycemic episodes and such symptoms as fatigue, shakiness, heart palpitations, and irritability. Researchers have also suggested that the rapid rise in insulin after you eat sugar may indirectly cause you to retain sodium and water.

Since sugar is a carbohydrate, and carbohydrates raise serotonin levels in the brain, some scientists have suggested that eating foods high in simple sugars would lead to nervous tension, drowsiness, and an inability to concentrate. As you have already seen, preliminary evidence from Dr. Wurtman's laboratory suggests that just the opposite happens: women with PMS feel calmer, more alert, and less depressed after eating high-carbohydrate foods (complex carbohydrates, that is).

This is not to say that you should load up on sugary foods to chase the blues away. Remember, the research suggesting that carbohydrates may improve your mood is too preliminary to make such blanket statements. Keep in mind, too, that the calories supplied by sugar and sweetened foods are largely "empty calories;" that is, the calories in these foods provide few of the vitamins and minerals your body needs to function. What's more, many foods made with large amounts of added sugar in them, such as cakes, pies, cookies, ice cream, and sweet rolls, also contain a hefty amount of fat. A high-fat diet has been associated with obesity, heart disease, and certain types of cancer.

Although it's probably not necessary to avoid sugar altogether during the premenstrual phase of your menstrual cycle, there are more healthful sources of carbohydrates than sugary foods—namely complex carbohydrates, such as pasta, rice, potatoes, foods made from whole grains, fruits, vegetables, and legumes (dried peas and beans). If you crave an occasional candy bar, it probably won't hurt to indulge now and then. But try to eat sugary foods along with other foods; it is less taxing on your blood sugar levels.

FAT

Certain fatty acids in the body are precursors of prostaglandins, and recommendations to cut back on animal fats (meat, milk, and dairy products) are based on the idea that diets high in animal fats may increase the body's production of prostaglandins that aggravate premenstrual symptoms. Animal fats contain the fatty acid *arachidonic acid*, which is a precursor of prostaglandins E_2 and $F_2\alpha$. These prostaglandins are believed to lower levels of another prostaglandin, E_1, causing an imbalance that theoretically could lead to increased premenstrual symptoms. Arachidonic acid is also a precursor of *leukotrienes* and other compounds believed to cause inflammation of the breast and other tissues.

No studies have shown that reducing your intake of fat—particularly saturated fats—will reduce premenstrual symptoms. Nevertheless, there are numerous other compelling reasons to cut back on fat and saturated fat in your diet. As we mentioned earlier, a high-fat diet has been associated with obesity, and an increased risk of heart disease and certain types of cancer, including breast cancer, one of the leading causes of cancer death among women. Indeed, the United States government, the American Heart Association, the American Cancer Association and other national health organizations now recommend that *all* Americans reduce their fat intake to no more than 30 percent of their total daily calories—PMS or no PMS.

One of the best ways to cut back on fat is to reduce your intake of foods high in fat, and meat and dairy products happen to be the two major sources of fat in our diets. This essentially means that you should

- Eat smaller portions of meat (two 3-ounce servings per day, together with protein from milk and dairy products is all most women really need);
- Choose leaner meats, such as fish, poultry with the skin removed, veal, and beef round and sirloin;
- Trim the visible fat off meat before cooking;
- Cook with the least amount of fat (broiling, braising and stewing are best; pan-frying and deep frying are less desirable);
- Choose low-fat and no-fat milk and dairy products.

When you cut back on fatty foods, you may find yourself losing weight (since fatty foods are also some of the most fattening—literally), and if you have high cholesterol, your cholesterol levels may improve. But it remains to be seen whether you'll see an improvement in your premenstrual symptoms.

PROTEIN

Some experts recommend that you eat more protein-rich foods to avoid episodes of hypoglycemia. Others say you should cut back on foods high in protein—particularly animal proteins, such as meat and milk—because excessive intake of animal protein is believed to stimulate prolactin, insulin, and luteinizing hormone secretions, all of which, some researchers say, leads to increased premenstrual symptoms. Another argument against eating too much protein is that protein contains large amounts of the amino acid *tyrosine*, which competes with tryptophan (the amino acid precursor of serotonin) for entry into the brain. Once tyrosine enters the brain, it increases levels of dopamine and norepinephrine, two neurotransmitters that make you feel more alert. At the same time, tryptophan levels fall, decreasing the brain's production of serotonin and its calming effect. And the two main sources of protein in the average American diet—meat and dairy products—also contain large amounts of saturated fat, which some scientists believe may also contribute to premenstrual symptoms (see "Fat," above).

Dr. Judith Wurtman's research suggests that women with PMS naturally avoid high protein foods. Since most Americans eat much more protein than they need, it certainly doesn't hurt to cut back. But again, there is no solid evidence that doing so will reduce your premenstrual symptoms.

CAFFEINE

Women with PMS are frequently advised to cut back on caffeine, a substance in coffee, tea, a variety of soft drinks, certain foods, and many over-the-counter and prescription medications. Annette MacKay Rossignol, head of Oregon State University's Department of Public Health reported in 1990 that consumption of caffeine-containing beverages is strongly related to the prevalence and severity of premenstrual symptoms, including depression, irritability, anxiety, headaches, and breast swelling and tenderness. Most other studies on the subject have suggested that the more caffeine you consume, the worse your symptoms are likely to be. Unfortunately, many of the women in these studies didn't meet the rigorous National Institutes of Mental Health criteria for having premenstrual syndrome, so the question of whether caffeine influences premenstrual symptoms is still up in the air.

So far, no studies have clearly shown that cutting back on caffeine will reduce the severity of your symptoms either. (Most researchers won't even attempt such a study since it is almost impossible to control a person's eating habits or accurately measure her caffeine consumption.) Nevertheless, it's probably a worthwhile experiment to cut back on caffeine for a few months and see if your symptoms improve, particularly since caffeine is not exactly a substance with much redeeming nutritional value. In fact, caffeine isn't a nutrient at all; technically, it is a food additive. And most foods (chocolate) and beverages (coffee, tea, cola, and other soft drinks) containing caffeine consist mainly of fat and sugar and not much else.

Caffeine is such a potent central nervous system stimulant that it is considered an "active ingredient" in many over-the-counter and prescription drugs. The substance has been known to trigger panic and anxiety attacks in affected people. And since many women with premenstrual symptoms also suffer from underlying emotional disorders, such as anxiety, it's better to be safe and stay away from this potential trigger.

Many caffeine-containing foods and beverages also contain *methylxanthines*, chemicals believed to exacerbate breast tenderness—at least among women with benign breast disease (also known as fibrocystic breast condition). Some women with fibrocystic breast condition report a reduction in pain, tenderness, and lumpiness when they reduce their intake of methylxanthines and a return of these symptoms when they increase their intake of these chemicals.

You may want to try cutting caffeine out of your diet altogether for at least two menstrual cycles before deciding whether the change is truly beneficial to you. If you find after this time that your symptoms are no better, there's no reason not to enjoy your morning brew. While in the recent past, concerns had been raised that caffeine might raise your risk of heart disease and fibrocystic breast condition or cause birth defects when consumed during pregnancy, the substance has largely been cleared of any wrongdoing. And although some questions still remain about its overall effect on your health, caffeine is one of 700 substances listed with the United States Food and Drug Administration as "generally recognized as safe" (GRAS)—when consumed in moderation, that is.

HOW TO REDUCE YOUR CAFFEINE INTAKE

Caffeine is found in literally hundreds of foods, beverages and over-the-counter medications—including some premenstrual formulas and diuretics (caffeine has diuretic properties). Each tablet of the diuretic Aquaban, for instance, contains 200 mg of caffeine—the equivalent of about two cups of coffee. Obviously, the first step in cutting back is to know which foods, beverages, and medications are high in caffeine (see

"Caffeine Content of Some Common Foods, Beverages, and Drugs," next page). This is an incomplete list, so be sure to read the labels of soft drinks and over-the-counter medications to see if they contain caffeine.

If you consume caffeine on a regular basis—a morning cup of coffee, for instance, or a cola with your lunch—and especially if you consume a lot of it, you can expect to experience such withdrawal symptoms as irritability, nervousness, restlessness, lethargy, nausea, and headaches when you stop, particularly if you quit cold turkey. To avoid these withdrawal symptoms, you should gradually wean yourself off the caffeine habit. For instance, if you drink three or more cups of coffee per day, drop down to two cups of coffee for a few days. After you've adjusted to two cups, gradually reduce your daily intake a quarter cup at a time to one cup and finally to none. Or switch to a half-caffeinated, half-decaffeinated brew and gradually increase the amount of decaffeinated coffee you use until your brew is 100 percent decaffeinated. Switch to decaffeinated soft-drinks and herbal teas, as well. Better yet, instead of a soft drink, have sparkling water, juice, or a juice spritzer (one-half juice, one-half sparkling water). Most juices contain at least some vitamins, while soft drinks have none.

CAFFEINE CONTENT OF SOME COMMON FOODS, BEVERAGES, AND DRUGS

Item	Caffeine (mg)
Coffee, 5-ounce cup	
Brewed, drip method	115
Instant	65
Decaffeinated, brewed	3
Decaffeinated, instant	2
Tea, 5-ounce cup	
U.S. brands, brewed	40
Imported brands, brewed	60
Instant	30
Iced (12-ounce glass)	70
Chocolate	
Cocoa beverage, 5-ounce cup	4
Chocolate milk, 8-ounce glass	5
Milk chocolate, 1 ounce	6
Dark, semisweet chocolate, 1 ounce	20
Soft drinks	
Cola or Pepper	30–45
Decaffeinated cola	trace–0.18
Caffeine-free cola	0
Orange	0
Other citrus*	0–54
Ginger ale, root beer, tonic water, soda, seltzer, sparkling water	0
Prescription Drugs	
Cafergot (for migraine headaches)	100
Fiorinal (for tension headaches)	40
Darvon Compound, pain reliever	32.4
Over-the-Counter Drugs**	
Analgesic/Pain Relief	
Anacin and Anacin Maximum Strength	32
Excedrin	65
Midol	32.4
Vanquish	33
Diuretics	
Aqua-Ban	200
Permathene H_2Off	200

*Soft drinks containing caffeine are so labeled.
**More than 100 over-the-counter drug products contain caffeine. Caffeine is often found in weight control aids, alertness tablets, headache and pain relief remedies, cold products, and diuretics. When caffeine is an ingredient, it is listed on the label.
Source: United States Food and Drug Administration, October, 1983.

COMPLEX CARBOHYDRATES

Whole grain foods, fruits, vegetables, legumes, and nuts and seeds are known in nutrition circles as *complex carbohydrates*. These foods generally are low in fat and high in vitamins, minerals, and fiber and—according to some nutrition surveys—are conspicuously absent from the diets of many women with PMS. Some researchers suggest that women with PMS may suffer from nutritional deficiencies precisely because they don't eat these nutrient-rich foods. And those who believe that sugar, fat, and protein may contribute to premenstrual symptoms recommend that women replace these foods with complex carbohydrates.

Remember, the surveys on which these recommendations are based may not be a true reflection of the diets of all women with PMS. So far, the best evidence suggesting that complex carbohydrates may help alleviate premenstrual symptoms comes from Dr. Judith Wurtman's study. And as well designed as it was, the study group didn't eat a "placebo" meal for comparison, so it can't be considered a placebo-controlled, double blind study—the gold standard by which most treatments for PMS are measured.

But because complex carbohydrates pack such a nutritional punch, you simply can't go wrong with the recommendation to eat more of these foods. Complex carbohydrates should be at the top of your grocery list whether or not you have PMS—and even if later studies don't support Dr. Wurtman's preliminary results.

VITAMINS AND MINERALS

Multivitamin and mineral supplements are some of the most widely used treatments for PMS today. But do they work?

And are they safe? Let's look at the evidence for individual vitamins and minerals first.

VITAMIN B₆

This vitamin, also known as *pyridoxine*, first received attention in the 1940s, when animal studies suggested that a deficiency of vitamin B_6 increases the breakdown of estrogen in the body, leading to lower estrogen levels. Later research has found that even women with a severe vitamin B deficiency don't have lower blood estrogen levels, and this theory has pretty much been abandoned.

Interest in vitamin B_6 as a possible remedy for premenstrual depression was revived when women taking oral contraceptives were found to experience mild deficiencies in vitamin B_6, and vitamin B_6 supplements were found to improve the mood of depressed oral contraceptive users. Vitamin B_6 is instrumental in the manufacture of several neurotransmitters in the brain, including dopamine and serotonin, and vitamin B_6 supplements are believed to fight the depression associated with oral contraceptive use by raising brain levels of serotonin and dopamine.

Other scientists have suggested that low levels of dopamine and serotonin (possibly induced by a vitamin B_6 deficiency) lead to high levels of prolactin and aldosterone, which could explain fluid retention associated with PMS. So in theory, vitamin B_6 supplements could prove beneficial in the treatment of PMS both as a natural diuretic and an antidepressant.

Dr. Guy Abraham reported in 1982 that the diets of some women with PMS contained less than half the recommended dietary allowance (2 to 4 mg per day) of vitamin B_6. So far, however, there is no direct evidence that women with PMS suffer from even mild vitamin B_6 deficiencies. And studies involving the use of vitamin B_6 in the treatment of premenstrual symptoms have been contradictory. Some have found that premenstrual depression and other symptoms improve among women who take vitamin B_6 supplements, while others have found no changes in the women's symptoms. In the studies that showed improved symptoms, the benefits of vitamin B_6 were not limited to the premenstrual phase of the cycle, suggesting that the supplement may have an overall effect on your mood and not necessarily a specific effect on PMS-associated depression.

Before you begin taking vitamin B_6, you should know that it is not without side effects. Although it was long believed that taking large doses of water soluble vitamins was safe because the body simply secreted whatever it didn't use, this doesn't appear to be the case for vitamin B_6. In one 1984 study, women taking 2,000 to 6,000 mg of pyridoxine daily experienced such side effects as burning, shooting or tingling pains, and numbness in the hands and feet, clumsiness or an unsteady gait, a condition known as *sensory neuropathy*. Some women have reported experiencing these symptoms when taking as little as 50 mg of vitamin B_6 per day. Most women find that symptoms gradually improve after they stop taking vitamin B_6 supplements.

The current recommended daily allowance (RDA) of vitamin B_6 is 2 mg per day. The best food sources of vitamin B_6 are yeast, wheat germ, sunflower seeds, chicken, tuna, legumes, whole grain cereals, bananas, and oatmeal. If you decide to take a vitamin B_6 supplement, you should limit your dosage to 50 to 100 mg per day. You should reduce the dosage even further or stop taking the supplement altogether if you experience numbness or tingling sensations in your fingers or feet. It's also better to take vitamin B_6 as part of a B-complex or multivitamin and mineral supplement because both magnesium and riboflavin, another B vitamin, are required for the conversion of the inactive form of vitamin B_6 found in supplements to a biologically active form that your body can use.

MAGNESIUM

A magnesium deficiency could theoretically explain many of the cyclical symptoms of PMS. A magnesium deficiency is known to cause a depletion of the neurotransmitter dopamine in the brain, which could lead to depression. Magnesium is also instrumental in the secretion of the hormone insulin from the pancreas, which regulates blood-sugar levels. The mineral plays a role in the production of prostaglandins, too. Finally, magnesium is suspected of influencing the body's fluid balance system. A magnesium deficiency could increase levels of the hormone aldosterone, leading to increased fluid retention. Aldosterone in turn, causes you to excrete more magnesium in your urine, which could worsen the initial magnesium deficiency that caused you to retain water, creating a vicious cycle.

Interest in magnesium grew when, in a small 1982 nutrition survey, Dr. Abraham found that women with PMS consume a daily average of 100 mg of magnesium less than unaffected women, suggesting that women with PMS may not get enough magnesium in their diets. Perhaps more importantly, several researchers have found physical evidence of a magnesium deficiency in women suffering from PMS.

Based on this evidence, Italian gynecologist Fabio Faccinetti, M.D., decided to see whether women with PMS would benefit from taking magnesium supplements. For the first two menstrual cycles of the study, 28 women with PMS took either a placebo or 120 mg of magnesium three times a day (a total daily intake of 360 mg of magnesium) from the fifteenth day of their menstrual cycle until they started their periods. Then all women took magnesium supplements in the same way for two more menstrual cycles. Throughout the course of the study, the women filled out a standardized menstrual distress questionnaire to determine the effectiveness of the treatment. The researchers found that women taking magnesium experienced a significant improvement in mood swings and depression but not in any other symptoms associated with PMS. The researchers suggest that magnesium "may restore some unbalanced neurotransmitter activity responsible for premenstrual mood and behavioral changes."

The study was small and the researchers didn't include a comparison group of normal women in their study. Obviously, larger studies need to be conducted before it can be said with certainty that magnesium helps alleviate the mood swings and depression associated with PMS. Nevertheless, it wouldn't hurt to increase your intake of magnesium. The best food choices are nuts, legumes, cereal grains, and dark green vegetables. Seafood is another good source of magnesium. Most PMS supplements contain magnesium, but they usually also contain high levels of vitamin B_6 and other vitamins and minerals that you may or may not need or want to take, so check the label before you buy. Or look for supplements containing magnesium only.

You should be aware that magnesium and calcium compete with each other in the body (for instance, calcium stimulates muscle contractions while magnesium relaxes muscles), and an excessive calcium intake can induce signs of a magnesium deficiency. For this reason, the recommended calcium-to-magnesium ratio is two-to-one: in other words, you should consume roughly twice as much calcium as you do magnesium. Consuming more calcium than this may hinder your body's absorption of magnesium. The current RDA for magnesium—300 mg per day—is based on the RDA for calcium of 800 mg per day. But if you take calcium supplements (as many women are now encouraged to do to fend off the bone thinning disorder osteoporosis), you should match your increased calcium intake with an increase in magnesium so that your calcium-to-magnesium ratio is two-to-one. In other words, if you consume 1,500 mg of calcium per day, your magnesium intake should be more along the lines of 700 mg per day. Magnesium isn't toxic, even in high doses. But remember that taking in too much magnesium can interfere with your body's use of calcium. So don't overdo it. Limit your magnesium consumption to no more than 700 mg per day.

CALCIUM

Calcium is an important part of bone health, and during the last ten years, most women have been encouraged to increase their calcium intake to help prevent the crippling bone disorder osteoporosis. Unfortunately, calcium's role in exacerbating or relieving premenstrual symptoms isn't so cut and dry.

Proponents of reducing your calcium intake point out that dairy products and calcium interfere with magnesium absorption. Moreover, rat studies suggest that excess brain calcium may interfere with intellectual performance and cause behavioral problems. These findings have been echoed in studies involving girls being rehabilitated for chronic criminal behavior. When the diets of the chronic offenders were compared with a group of nondelinquent girls, only one significant difference was found: the chronic offenders consumed an average of 35 ounces of milk daily, compared with 17 ounces for the nondelinquent girls, suggesting that the high consumption of dairy products (which are high in calcium) led to aggressive behavior in these girls.

Contrary to this evidence, Baylor College of Medicine's C. James Chuong, M.D., found in 1992 that women with PMS had markedly *lower* blood calcium levels than unaffected women during the luteal phase of the menstrual cycle, suggesting that excessive calcium is *not* associated with premenstrual symptoms. And a 1992 study by United States Department of Agriculture researchers found that nine out of ten women with PMS experienced a significant improvement in their symptoms when they consumed a diet that included 1,300 mg of calcium daily.

It's a known fact that diets chronically low in calcium impair bone health. Until we know more about the effects of calcium on premenstrual syndrome, a prudent approach would be to keep your calcium *and* magnesium intake high and in balance; that is, maintain a calcium-to-magnesium ratio of two-to-one.

Milk and dairy products happen to be the best dietary sources of calcium. But as we mentioned earlier, whole milk and whole dairy products are also high in fat. So stick with low-fat or skim milk and low- and no-fat yogurt, ice milk, and low-fat cheeses, such as mozzarella made from skim milk.

Dairy products aren't the only foods high in calcium. Other excellent sources include oysters, clams, salmon (with bones), sardines, tofu, broccoli, collard, turnip and mustard greens, kale, almonds, peanuts, and blackstrap molasses. Calcium-fortified orange juice and bread are other good choices. Calcium supplements are perfectly acceptable alternatives.

VITAMIN E

Some researchers have proposed the idea that premenstrual symptoms may be aggravated or caused by a deficiency in vitamin E. Animal studies suggesting that vitamin E might be instrumental in the body's production of prostaglandins bolstered the theory. But to date, there's no solid scientific evidence proving that vitamin E supplements actually reduce premenstrual symptoms. A handful of studies have shown improvements in such physical symptoms as breast tenderness and bloating among women who took vitamin E. But most women in these studies didn't experience any improvement in such psychological symptoms as irritability, depression, tension, confusion, headaches, or food cravings. Moreover, critics point out that the researchers didn't use the rigorous criteria of the National Institute of

Mental Health to screen the women, so it's questionable whether some of the women in these studies even had PMS.

There's no proof that women with PMS actually suffer from a vitamin E deficiency, either. None of the women in the studies just mentioned were found to have a vitamin E deficiency. And in a 1990 study, Dr. C. James Chuong and colleagues at Baylor College of Medicine also didn't find any detectable vitamin E deficiencies among women with PMS and a comparison group of unaffected women in either the follicular or luteal phase of their menstrual periods.

Vitamin E is the most widely available of any of the vitamins. Wheat germ oil is the richest source of vitamin E, but other cereal germs, green plants, egg yolk, milk fat, butter, meat, nuts, and vegetable oils also contain vitamin E.

What about supplements? Vitamin E supplements are readily available and have been touted as a remedy for a number of ills, including heart disease, thrombophlebitis, fibrocystic breasts, muscular dystrophy, menstrual problems, and miscarriage. If you do decide to try vitamin E supplements, don't take more than 400 international units (I.U.) per day. Women who take more than 600 I.U. per day may experience a significant reduction in thyroid hormone and elevated blood triglyceride levels (a possible risk factor for heart disease). In addition, high levels of vitamin E may interfere with vitamin K in some people, possibly leading to bleeding problems. (Vitamin K is instrumental in the formation of blood clots.) If you take a specially formulated premenstrual vitamin and mineral supplement, check the label for the amount of vitamin E and other vitamins in the supplement.

VITAMIN A

In 1947, researchers using massive doses of vitamin A to treat women with hyperthyroidism incidentally discovered that the treatment "cured" the symptoms of PMS in one patient. Other researchers subsequently reported that 30 patients with PMS were successfully treated with 200,000 international units (IU) of vitamin A daily. The scientists suggested that vitamin A might correct a problem with estrogen metabolism in women with PMS, and that vitamin A might also act as a diuretic.

Before you swallow any claims about vitamin A as an aid for PMS, you should be aware that neither of these theories has been substantiated. Moreover, taking megadoses of vitamin A for an extended period of time can cause a toxic buildup of this oil-soluble vitamin in the liver, resulting in such symptoms as itching, hair loss, dry skin and mouth, irritability, nausea or vomiting, bone and joint pains, fatigue, and chronic headaches. Excessive amounts of vitamin A can also cause irreversible liver damage. Nevertheless, large and potentially dangerous amounts of vitamin A are sometimes prescribed for women with PMS and can still be found in many premenstrual multivitamin preparations.

The current recommended dietary allowance of vitamin A is 4,000 IU for women. If you eat a balanced diet, you will get all the vitamin A you need from such foods as dark green leafy vegetables, cantaloupe, carrots, sweet potatoes, and winter squash, which are high in *beta carotene,* a precursor that is converted into vitamin A by the body. Other foods high in vitamin A (retinol) are liver, fish oil, butter, and egg yolks. There is really no reason to take large doses of vitamin A or beta carotene for the treatment of PMS. If you do take supplements, choose those containing beta carotene rather than retinol. Beta carotene is nontoxic, even in high doses.

PREMENSTRUAL VITAMIN
AND MINERAL SUPPLEMENTS

Although there's no shortage of premenstrual vitamin and mineral supplements available to women, there is most definitely a shortage of double-blind, placebo-controlled studies to determine whether the supplements actually work. Dr. Guy Abraham did conduct one placebo-controlled, double-blind, crossover study on the nutritional supplement Optivite (manufactured by Dr. Abraham's own Optimox Corporation in Torrence, California). Each supplement contains high levels of vitamin B_6, magnesium, and vitamin A. Sixteen of the twenty-three women reported feeling better during the cycles in which they took Optivite, while only seven felt better when they took a placebo.

Most supplements contain high doses of vitamin B_6, magnesium, vitamin E, and vitamin A. And while there's little evidence that magnesium and vitamin E can be toxic at high doses, the same can't be said for vitamin B_6, which can cause nerve damage when taken in high doses. Vitamin A can build up to toxic levels in the liver when taken in high doses over an extended period of time.

EVENING PRIMROSE OIL

This nutritional supplement contains an oil from the seeds of the evening primrose flower, as well as vitamin E. The oil contains *gamma linoleic acid*, a saturated fat necessary for the body to manufacture prostaglandin E_1. Because prostaglandin imbalances are suspected of playing a role in PMS, some researchers have theorized that treating women with this prostaglandin precursor would help alleviate symptoms.

Early, uncontrolled studies showed a dramatic reduction in premenstrual symptoms among women who took evening primrose oil. However, more recent placebo-controlled studies have found that evening primrose oil is no more effective than placebo in relieving symptoms of PMS, with the exception, perhaps, of breast tenderness. One study has found that evening primrose oil is as good as the drug bromocriptine (Parlodel) in relieving breast tenderness and causes fewer side effects.

Evening primrose oil can be found in some health food stores but, technically, sale of the supplements in this country is illegal. According to the United States Food and Drug Administration, there just isn't enough data demonstrating the effectiveness of evening primrose oil to support the various health claims on the product label (including claims about improving premenstrual symptoms) made by the manufacturers of these supplements.

ALCOHOL

Of the estimated 2 million alcoholic women of reproductive age in the United States, 67 percent relate their drinking to their menstrual cycles. The highest reported number of drinking bouts usually occur during the premenstrual phase of the menstrual cycle. Apparently, many women turn to alcohol to relieve the anxiety and nervous tension just before menstruation.

Unfortunately, this is probably the worst time to reach for a drink to calm your nerves. There's evidence that fluctuations in hormones during the menstrual cycle affect the way you metabolize (break down) alcohol. Studies comparing blood-alcohol levels among women at various stages in the menstrual cycle show that the highest peaks in blood alcohol levels occur just before menstruation, suggesting that women are most vulnerable to alcohol's intoxicating effects at this time. Alcohol tends to lower blood sugar levels, too, possibly triggering or exacerbating hypoglycemic episodes at a time when you may already be vulnerable to low blood sugar levels. Alcohol is also a central nervous system depressant, and while it may initially lift your spirits and take the edge off nervous tension, when the effects of the drink wear off, you're likely to be stuck with an emotional hangover as well as a physical one. For this reason, you should find another, more constructive way to relax in the days just before your period (see Chapter 5 for suggestions).

IF YOU HAVE MENSTRUAL MIGRAINES

One group of women for whom dietary changes can often make a world of difference are those who suffer from menstrual migraines or a premenstrual worsening of their migraines. Certain foods can trigger migraine headaches, and avoiding these foods—particularly in the last part of your menstrual cycle when you are more vulnerable to migraine attacks—can often help prevent a debilitating headache. Some of the most offending substances include the following:

- Foods high in chemicals known as *amines* (including serotonin, tyramine, and norepinephrine). Bananas, pineapples, plums, tomatoes, and nuts contain high levels of serotonin. Aged cheeses, pickled herring, chicken liver, canned figs, sour cream, bananas, and some alcoholic beverages contain tyramine. Citrus fruits contain large amounts of L-octapamine (norsynephrine).
- Aspartame (Nutrasweet, Equal). After this sugar substitute was introduced in 1981, the United States Centers for Disease Control in Atlanta received a rash of complaints about headaches (as well as other symptoms) from people who consumed foods or beverages containing aspartame. Although subsequent studies have not confirmed that aspartame is a

migraine trigger, you should avoid this substance if
you get aspartame-related headaches.

- Monosodium glutamate (MSG). This food additive
  is commonly used to season Chinese food and a
  number of commercially processed foods, including
  many frozen foods (particularly dinner entrees),
  canned and dried soups, processed snacks, cured
  meats, packaged sauces, and prepared salad dress-
  ings. If you are sensitive to MSG, check the labels of
  processed and prepackaged foods before you buy
  them, and when eating in a Chinese restaurant,
  request that your food be prepared without MSG.
- Nitrates. This food preservative and coloring agent is
  commonly found in salami, baloney, pepperoni,
  ham, bacon, and hot dogs.
- Alcohol. Alcohol is a potent blood vessel constrictor
  and may in itself be a migraine trigger. Many alcoholic beverages, particularly red wines, also contain
  other known migraine triggers, such as sulfites.
- Caffeine. This substance constricts blood vessels and
  can often be used to abort a headache. But consuming too much caffeine may trigger a rebound
  headache. So use caffeine in moderation, if at all.
  (For a list of caffeine-containing foods and beverages, see page 73.)
- Erratic eating habits. Skipping meals, dieting, or fast-
  ing may trigger a headache, so try not to go more
  than four hours without eating.

You may not be susceptible to *all* of these potential
migraine triggers. To find out what sets off a headache in you,
keep a diary of your migraine attacks, recording the time of
onset and listing the foods you've eaten in the past twenty-four
hours. After a while, a pattern will begin to emerge, and you

and your physician should be able to identify the offending substance and avoid it.

As you can see, most of the dietary recommendations for women with PMS—reducing your intake of fat, refined sugars, white flour, coffee, tea, and chocolate, cutting back on your alcohol consumption and eating more complex carbohydrates, such as foods made from whole grains, fruits and vegetables, nuts, seeds, and legumes—make good nutritional sense regardless of whether or not you have PMS. And if following these dietary recommendations improves your premenstrual symptoms, so much the better!

Many women with mild to moderate premenstrual symptoms find that they do feel better and that their symptoms improve by making changes in their diets—particularly by reducing their intake of sodium, caffeine, and alcohol. Whether the therapeutic effects of the other recommendations come from the dietary changes themselves or simply from the sense of control you feel remains to be seen, but you have nothing to lose by trying the recommendations here. As for PMS vitamin and mineral supplements, use them at your own risk, and stay away from supplements containing megadoses of vitamins B_6 and A.

CHAPTER 5

MANAGING STRESS

Premenstrual symptoms are stressful in themselves. But when premenstrual tension is compounded by everyday stress, the combination can be particularly hard on you. This is why a general treatment regimen for PMS should include a strategy for managing stress.

WHAT IS STRESS?

Stress is actually a broad term used to describe stressors—any kind of change that requires you to adapt in one way or another. Stressors can be physical—a broken arm, which requires increased blood flow, nutrients, and plenty of rest to mend; or psychological—having to adjust to your relative inability to use your arm as it heals. Stress can be negative—losing your job or getting stuck in traffic; or positive—getting married or taking a vacation. Most of us use the term "stress" to describe the psychological stressors in our lives, and that's what we'll be talking about in this chapter.

Although most stressors today tax your emotions, your body responds in a very physical way—with what is known as the *fight or flight response*. This is an inborn trait that evolved hundreds of thousands of years ago to protect primitive peoples from such physical threats as wild animals. When the fight or flight response is triggered, your adrenal glands begin pumping out two related "stress hormones," *epinephrine* and *norepinephrine* (also sometimes referred to collectively as *adrenaline*). These hormones work on your sympathetic nervous system (the part of the central nervous system that affects such involuntary functions as your heart rate and breathing) and accelerate your breathing and pulse rate, raise your blood pressure, boost your blood-sugar levels, and release high-energy fats into the bloodstream, preparing you to fight off a physical threat or flee from it.

The fight-or-flight response served early peoples well. But it does little to help you cope with the psychological stressors of the modern-day world. And many experts now believe that the constant firing of the fight-or-flight response and the needless flooding of the body with these stress hormones could lead to a whole host of stress-related illnesses. Stress has been shown to make you more susceptible to the common cold, headaches, and minor gastrointestinal upsets. Mounting evidence now suggests that stress may play a role in the development of more serious illnesses, including heart disease, high blood pressure, arthritis, peptic ulcers, and possibly cancer.

In addition, stress can worsen existing medical conditions, including PMS. For instance, some researchers have documented increased mood swings, pain, and water retention among women with PMS who are simultaneously going through a divorce, loss of a job, or other "negative life changes." Moreover, premenstrual tension can heighten your response to everyday stressors and minor annoyances that might not otherwise bother you. Indeed, there's some evidence to suggest that women experience an exaggerated response to stress during the last half of the menstrual cycle, including an increased heart rate and blood pressure and higher levels of epinephrine and norepinephrine.

A PROGRAM FOR MANAGING
PREMENSTRUAL STRESS

Stress is an inevitable part of life, the natural consequence of change. You can't escape it. But you can change the way you respond to it.

Apparently, having a sense of control (either real or imagined) is an important part of managing stress. A 1988 study by psychiatrist Alan Breier, M.D., and colleagues at the National Institute of Mental Health in Bethesda illustrates just how important having a sense of control is in terms of reducing stress. The researchers subjected ten healthy volunteers to a loud, irritating noise while they took a word-scramble test on two separate days. When the volunteers could stop the noise by pressing a sequence of buttons in front of them, their elevated levels of stress hormones fell almost immediately after the noise stopped. When the buttons no longer worked and the volunteers *couldn't* stop the noise, their stress hormones remained elevated for as long as forty-five minutes after the word test ended.

Suzanne Kobasa, Ph.D., and colleagues at the City University of New York have found that people who weather stress better than others appear to have "stress hearty" personalities, characterized by an attitude of commitment in their approach to work and life, a take-charge approach to life events rather than a passive acceptance, and the view that adversity and conflict are opportunities for personal growth rather than threats to be escaped. How can *you* manage?

WHAT YOU CAN DO

If these studies are any indication, virtually everything you do about your PMS—reading up on the condition, seeking professional help, charting your symptoms—can help give you a sense of control over your condition. Here are a few other ways to help take the edge off everyday stress and tension and help you feel more in control.

Exercise

Exercise is a natural muscle-relaxant and overall tension reliever. Regular, aerobic exercises that raise your heart rate and breathing—walking, jogging, running, stair-climbing, swimming, bicycling, or aerobic dance—help clear the stress hormones epinephrine and norepinephrine from your body by putting them to their intended use. What's more, when you exercise, your body produces and releases a group of hormones known as *beta endorphins*—the same hormones that produce feelings of euphoria experienced by long-distance runners, known as the "runner's high." When you've finished your workout, you're left in a state of natural relaxation. Your heart rate decreases, your blood pressure declines, and your breathing slows down. Your muscles are more relaxed, too. Exercise can even help ease your mind of excessive worry, as your concentration shifts to your workout instead of the hassles of the day.

Two small studies by Jerilynn Prior, M.D., and colleagues at the University of British Columbia in Vancouver have suggested that exercise may even help relieve certain premenstrual symptoms. In 1986, the researchers enlisted eight sedentary women to run an average of thirty-two miles per menstrual cycle. After three months, the women reported significantly less breast discomfort and swelling than a comparison group of six sedentary women. In a 1987 study lasting six months, eight other volunteers who ran an average of forty-seven miles per cycle again reported less breast tenderness, swelling, and anxiety than six ordinarily active women who were not in training.

There's also indirect evidence that exercise can help relieve premenstrual symptoms. Exercise has been shown to reduce symptoms in depressive illness. And women who exercise have fewer symptoms in the luteal phase of the menstrual cycle than women who do not exercise. Too, as we pointed out earlier, exercise boosts endorphin activity in the brain, which could conceivably help counteract the drop in endorphin activity before menstruation.

It would be premature to promise that exercise will relieve your premenstrual symptoms based on these studies and the indirect evidence. Both of Dr. Prior's studies were small, and there's no way to measure the effectiveness of exercise against a placebo. Nevertheless, because of its natural ability to relieve tension, as well as a host of other health benefits (including a reduced risk of heart disease, hypertension, cancer, diabetes, and osteoporosis), exercise should be an integral part of any PMS management program.

If you've been sedentary for more than a year—particularly if you are over age forty—you should check with your doctor first before launching an exercise program. Once you've been given the okay to exercise, you should carefully consider which activity (or activities) would best suit your needs. Aerobic exercises work best for reducing stress. Be sure to choose an activity that you enjoy doing, and one that is convenient for you; this helps increase compliance. One of the easiest, most enjoyable activities for most women is brisk walking, as it doesn't require any special equipment and you can walk practically anywhere—even in an indoor shopping mall (provided, of course, you don't stop to window shop!). Walking is also less likely to result in injury, since it is a low-impact activity.

Once you've decided on an activity, make a time commitment to exercise. Block off some time for your exercise sessions in your appointment book and honor these appointments with yourself as you would any other appointment with a professional or business associate.

Whatever activity you choose, be sure to start out slowly—perhaps just five or ten minutes per day, five or six days a week in the first weeks of training. This helps to gradually condition your body to increased activity, ease muscle soreness that often plagues beginners, and reduce the risk of sustaining an exercise-related injury. Short, frequent exercise sessions also help make a habit of exercising—a habit that hopefully you won't want to give up.

Over the next three to six weeks, you'll want to work up to longer exercise sessions that raise your heart rate to a working level—about 60 to 80 percent of its maximum capacity—for at least twenty to thirty minutes. You can calculate your working heart range using the following equation:

$$220 - \text{your age} \times .60 \text{ to } .80$$

So if you are thirty-three years old, you would calculate your target heart range as follows:

$$220 - 33 = 187 \times .60 \text{ to } .80 = 112 \text{ to } 149$$

In other words, your target heart range would be between 112 and 149 beats per minute.

Now calculate your own target heart range here:

$$220 - (\text{your age}) \times .60 = \underline{\hspace{1.5cm}}$$
$$\times .80 = \underline{\hspace{1.5cm}}$$

Periodically taking your pulse during your workout will help you determine whether or not you are exercising strenuously enough to raise your heart rate to this level. To take your pulse, place the index and middle fingers (not your thumb) of your right hand over the carotid artery on the left side of your neck. Using a watch with a second hand or a digital watch that shows seconds, count your pulse for ten seconds and multiply the number of pulse beats you counted by six. Your pulse beats should fall somewhere within your target heart range.

When you have PMS, there are bound to be days when you feel so down or physically uncomfortable that you simply don't want to exercise. Berating yourself for not exercising won't make you feel any better. Rather, ease up on yourself and do whatever amount of exercise you feel up to; for instance, if you don't have the energy to jog a mile or two, walk instead. If you are tired of walking, take a short bike ride. The important thing is to try to engage in some kind of physical activity so you don't lose momentum. Remember, too that the times when you feel your worst are the times that you most need the stress-relieving benefits of exercise. After you've finished exercising, reward yourself with a small treat—a movie or a new pair of earrings, for example. Even if you don't exercise for a day or two, tell yourself that "tomorrow is another day," and start exercising again as soon as you are able.

On days when you're plagued with lower backache and other premenstrual and menstrual aches and pains, you may find some relief with a few simple stretches. Try the stretches here (see Figures 6 through 9) to help relieve lower-back tension.

Relaxation Exercises

Relaxation techniques—yoga, deep breathing, progressive muscle relaxation, and meditation, to name a few—help elicit what Harvard University cardiologist Herbert Benson, M.D., calls the "relaxation response," a state of consciousness marked by decreased oxygen consumption, respiratory rate, heart rate, and blood pressure. Physiologically, the relaxation response is the exact opposite of what happens during the stress-induced fight-or-flight response.

The relaxation response has been shown to help lower blood pressure among people with hypertension, and there's some evidence that relaxation exercises may permanently decrease your body's response to the stress hormone norepinephrine. Working with Dr. Benson, Irene Goodale, Ph.D., has also found that the relaxation response may help improve emotional symptoms among women with PMS. In a five-month study of 107 women conducted at Harvard Medical School in 1990, those who elicited the relaxation response for 15 to 20 minutes every day experienced a significant reduction in such symptoms as hostility, irritability, anger, and anxiety. Fifty-eight percent of the women with the most severe symptoms experienced a decrease in their symptoms when they practiced the relaxation response, compared with 17 percent of women who only charted their symptoms. The researchers speculate that the relaxation response may help reduce premenstrual tension by decreasing your responsiveness to norepinephrine, which is believed to influence such moods and behaviors as aggression and anxiety.

Again, this was not a placebo-controlled study, but the results are encouraging. And it certainly can't hurt to try. After all, what have you got to lose but ten to twenty minutes per day spent in a state of relaxed tranquility?

How to Elicit the Relaxation Response

- Sit quietly in a comfortable position.
- Close your eyes.
- Deeply relax all your muscles.
- Breathe in and out through your nose; repeat the number "one" silently. This helps clear your mind of extraneous thoughts.
- Continue this routine for ten to twenty minutes.
- When finished, sit quietly with your eyes closed for a few moments, then gradually open them.

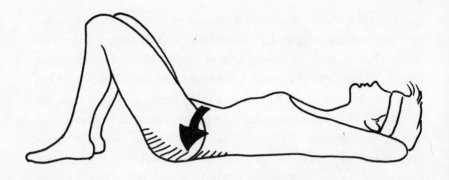

FIGURE 6 Pelvic tilt. With your hands behind your head, your knees bent, and your feet flat on the floor, tighten the muscles of your buttocks and abdomen, flattening your back against the floor. Hold the position for 5 to 10 seconds, then relax. Repeat the exercise two to three times.

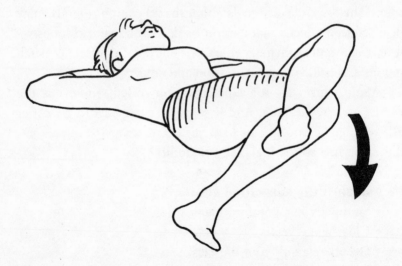

FIGURE 7 Crossed-leg stretch. With your hands behind your head, cross your left leg over your right leg and pull your right leg to the floor until you feel a stretch along the side of the hip and in the lower back (your right knee does not have to touch the floor). Keep the back of your head, your elbows, shoulders, and upper back flat on the floor. Hold the stretch for 10 to 30 seconds. Repeat the stretch on the other side. If you don't feel a stretch, create more muscle tension by holding down the right leg with the left leg as you try to pull the right leg back to an upright position.

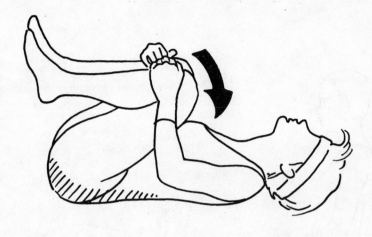

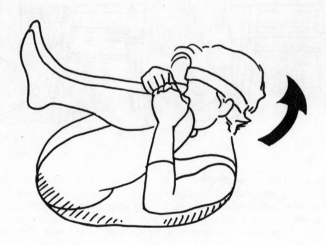

FIGURE 8 Knee-to-chest stretch. Pull both knees to your chest, keeping the back of your head down. Now curl your head toward your knees. Hold for 10 to 30 seconds and lower your head back down to the floor. Repeat the stretch three times.

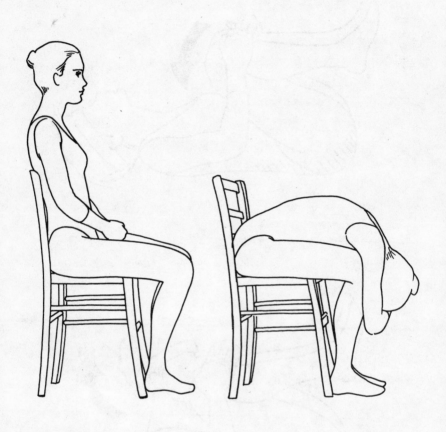

FIGURE 9 Chair stretch. Sit on a straight-back chair facing straight ahead (left). Fold your arms loosely on your lap and drop forward until your head is between your knees, letting your arms slide forward toward your ankles (right). Hold the stretch for 10 to 30 seconds. Tighten your abdominal muscles while returning to the starting position. Repeat the exercise three times.

Reduce Stress at Home and in the Office

You should make your life as easy as possible during the premenstrual phase of your menstrual cycle. This means keeping your personal and professional commitments to a minimum and building more personal time into your schedule.

Educating your friends, family members, and co-workers about your condition helps, too. Chances are good that family, friends, and co-workers are just as bewildered by your premenstrual personality changes as you are. With a clear understanding of the problem, the people closest to you will be better able to offer support during your premenstrual days.

Join a Support Group

It's often an enormous relief to know that others feel the same way you do. For this reason, you may want to join a PMS support group. To find one in your area, check your local newspaper (most provide a listing of various support groups), ask your doctor, or call local hospitals and women's health clinics. Check the Recommended Resources on page 144 for the names of a few national PMS support networks that may also be of help.

WHAT A PROFESSIONAL CAN DO

Exercise, relaxation exercises, and educating those around you about your condition can only go so far in alleviating stress. Unfortunately, for women with moderate to severe PMS, these measures often don't go far enough. Remember: it's not so much the stressors in your life as it is the way you respond to them that makes your life stressful. Therefore, making lasting changes in the way you respond to stress is essential for the long-term success of your treatment program.

Changing your behavior is not easy. For this reason, most women with PMS can benefit immensely by working closely with a psychologist, psychiatrist, or other mental health professional. Indeed, when Lorraine Dennerstein, M.D., and colleagues at the University of Melbourne in Australia compared the effectiveness of behavioral therapy, drug therapy (progesterone), and relaxation exercises in relieving premenstrual symptoms, they found significant reductions in anger, anxiety, irritability, and depression among women who received training in coping skills by a professional. Moreover, the improvements lasted throughout the course of the three-month study and for at least three months after the study officially ended. The positive responses to drug therapy and relaxation exercises wore off after the first two months of the study.

Many women feel perfectly comfortable seeing a therapist. If you've never been to a mental health professional, however, you may balk at the idea of seeing one. You may say to yourself, "I don't need a psychiatrist. I don't have a mental illness." You may even take your doctor's recommendation that you see a therapist as proof positive that he or she thinks your problem is "all in your head." Unless you are seeing a doctor who doesn't believe in PMS (yes, there are a few out there), your physician's suggestion that you see a mental health professional is simply his or her way of helping you both physically *and* emotionally. By referring you to a psychologist or other qualified counselor, your physician is recognizing his or her own limitations in treating your condition.

Unfortunately, negative attitudes about mental health professional are pervasive in our society—largely because of the stigma associated with mental illness. Because we know so little about so many disorders of the mind, and because the most serious mental illnesses—schizophrenia, paranoia, personality disorders, and the like—often evoke bizarre behavior and may even require institutionalization, most of us would rather keep a safe distance from anything that could be even remotely associated with mental illness—including a few sessions with a counselor or therapist. Indeed, this stigma associated with mental illness is precisely why many women were in an uproar after premenstrual syndrome (late luteal phase distrophic disorder, to be exact) was listed in the *Diagnostic and Statistical Manual of Mental Disorders-III* (DSM-III) as a "Diagnostic Category Needing Further Study."

You don't have to be mentally ill to benefit from the counseling and advice of a mental health professional. In fact, the people who benefit most are often those with less serious emotional problems—like PMS.

A counselor can help you break up the logjam of negative behavior patterns that may have evolved over the years between you and your loved ones or co-workers, particularly those patterns arising from your PMS. One of your counselor's jobs is to help make you more aware of these negative behavioral or communications patterns, and to help you break the cycle by suggesting alternative behaviors or ways of communicating your thoughts and feelings. These suggestions may be as simple as offering more effective ways of getting a point across to your spouse, children, or colleagues at work. Another role of the counselor is a hand-holder, offering reassurance, support and—if necessary—a shoulder to cry on as you experiment with new ways of responding to old stressors.

Overall, a counselor or therapist (there are many different kinds; see "How to Find a Counselor," below) can boost your self-esteem, help you work out the kinks in your personal and professional relationships, and generally help put your life back in order. So why not give counseling a try?

How to Find a Counselor

Since the best results come when you work with someone with whom you feel comfortable enough to share your innermost thoughts and feelings, you'll want to choose a counselor carefully. Begin by familiarizing yourself with the various types of counselors available to you.

PSYCHIATRISTS

These professionals have completed four years of medical school and three additional years of training in a psychiatric residency school. If you suffer from underlying depression or anxiety in addition to PMS, you may want to consider seeing a psychiatrist, as they are the only therapists who can prescribe drugs. (Antidepressants and other psychotropic drugs combined with counseling can be highly effective against these emotional disorders.) The psychiatrist should be licensed to practice in your state and may be certified by the American Board of Psychiatry and Neurology. If you have medical insurance, the fees of a psychiatrist are likely to be reimbursed.

CLINICAL PSYCHOLOGISTS

These professionals have Ph.D. degrees in psychology plus at least one year of supervised clinical training. They must pass a state licensing examination to practice, and their services are often covered by medical insurance. They may be certified by the American Board of Examiners in Professional Psychology.

SOCIAL WORKERS

These professionals generally hold master's degrees, although some have Ph.D. degrees, as well. They have completed at least two years of graduate study and two years of clinical internship. Many social workers are employed by hospitals and clinics, but some have private practices. They may or may not be eligible for insurance payments.

MENTAL HEALTH COUNSELORS

Some counselors hold master's degrees or Ed.S. degrees from graduate programs in education. Others with degrees in psychiatric nursing are also trained to counsel.

If you are unsure of the type of counselor you should see, ask your physician. If you haven't already had a psychological evaluation as part of your diagnostic work-up, you may also want to ask your doctor for a referral. Friends or relatives may be able to recommend a counselor, as well.

While it's important that the counselor you choose have a graduate education in counseling and supervised training, ultimately, the expertise and skill of the individual counselor may be more critical than a specific degree. For this reason, it's a good idea to interview one or more counselors before making a decision. At the initial visit, ask about the counselor's theories of counseling and whether short- or long-term counseling is used. Ask about fees and insurance coverage, too.

HOW NOT TO RELAX

Although you may be tempted to take the edge off premenstrual nervous tension with a stiff drink, yet another cup of coffee, or (if you smoke) a cigarette, these substances will only add to your problem. According to the National Institute of Alcohol Abuse and Alcoholism, you're likely to feel stronger effects from a given amount of alcohol when you're emotionally upset or under stress than you would when drinking the same amount while you are relaxed. This effect is likely to be compounded during the premenstrual phase of your menstrual cycle, when women are generally more susceptible to the intoxicating effects of alcohol. And research has shown that you're more likely to experience a more severe hangover during a time of stress than you would otherwise.

As we mentioned in Chapter 4, caffeine is a powerful central nervous system stimulant, which intensifies the effects of stress on the sympathetic nervous system. The nicotine in cigarettes has the same effect.

So instead of having a drink, a cup of coffee, or a cigarette, try taking a brisk walk or a bicycle ride. Or spend the time you would normally take to make yourself a drink or smoke a cigarette in quiet meditation instead.

CHAPTER 6

DRUG THERAPIES

Most women with severe PMS will require some sort of drug therapy to help alleviate their symptoms. Depending on the type and severity of your symptoms, your physician may recommend one of two general approaches: if you have just one or two particularly bothersome symptoms, such as breast tenderness and bloating, you may benefit from medication prescribed to help relieve those specific symptoms, what we call *symptomatic therapy*. Women with a variety of symptoms, including severe depression, may find relief from medications that alter their entire reproductive hormonal pattern, what we refer to as *syndromal therapy*.

For the most part, the medications used in the treatment of PMS are safe and effective. You should be aware, however, that not all drugs are equally effective in all women. You and your doctor may have to experiment with a few different medications before finding the right one for you. Keep in mind, too, that most medications will *improve* your symptoms, not cure them.

Here's a look at some of the available medications for the treatment of PMS.

SYMPTOMATIC THERAPY

If you have one or two dominant symptoms, you may be helped by one of the treatment approaches here.

FLUID RETENTION, BLOATING

These are some of the most common premenstrual symptoms, even though there is no experimental evidence that women with PMS actually retain fluid. Most women find that the problem can be adequately managed by cutting back on sodium (see page 64). Calcium and/or magnesium supplements may help, too.

If these measures don't work and especially if your symptoms chart reveals a premenstrual weight gain, your doctor may recommend that you use a diuretic. These drugs work by increasing the kidneys' excretion of salt and water. There are many types of diuretics, each of which affects a different part of the kidney. *Loop* and *thiazide diuretics*, used mainly in the treatment of heart disease and hypertension, are not normally recommended for women with PMS because, when taken cyclically, they may raise levels of the water-retaining hormone aldosterone and produce a "rebound" effect, causing you to regain water weight after you stop taking them. The same is true of over-the-counter "water pills," such as Aquaban and Diurex, and PMS and menstrual products (Midol and Pamprin) containing the active ingredient pamabrom or ammonium chloride.

Because of this rebound effect, many women who use these drugs find themselves in an upward spiral of diuretic abuse, taking more and more diuretics to offset the water weight gain that occurs when they stop taking the medications. (If you already suffer from a diuretic dependency, see "Breaking the Chain of Diuretic Abuse," page 107.) Women with PMS are particularly vulnerable, because they tend to take diuretics for a week or so, then stop taking them. For this reason, your physician will prescribe one of the milder *potassium-sparing* diuretics, such as *spironolactone* (Aldactone, and available in a generic form), *triamterene* (Dyrenium) and *amiloride* (Midamor, and available in a generic form). These diuretics are less likely to trigger the rebound effect associated with other types of diuretics and, therefore, they are safer to take cyclically. Spironolactone may be particularly useful for PMS, since it counters the water-retaining effects of the hormone aldosterone, (see Figure 10, page 117), which is suspected of causing fluid retention associated with PMS.

As with all medications, potassium-sparing diuretics may cause some side effects, including confusion, irregular heartbeat, numbness, or tingling in the hands, feet, or lips, shortness of breath, nervousness, or fatigue (these are signs of *hyperkalemia*, or higher-than-normal potassium levels).

If you do use diuretics, you will probably notice a reduction in premenstrual bloating and swelling. But there's little evidence that diuretics can relieve mood swings, depression, irritability, and other emotional symptoms. Indeed, in one study comparing the effectiveness of a mild diuretic with lithium (a drug used in the treatment of manic-depressive illness) and a placebo, the placebo was found to be the most effective in relieving emotional symptoms, followed by the diuretic. So don't expect more from these drugs than they can deliver.

BREAKING THE CHAIN OF DIURETIC ABUSE

When you take diuretics for more than a few days, your kidneys begin reducing the amount of sodium excreted in the urine in an effort to keep sodium levels in the body from dropping too low. (Sodium helps maintain the body's fluid and electrolyte balance and is instrumental in nerve impulse transmission). So, in effect, the drugs help program the kidneys to hold onto sodium, which causes you to regain water weight when you stop taking them.

If you are already "hooked" on diuretics, how can you break the cycle? Know first that you can expect some weight gain when you stop taking diuretics—a few pounds, on average. For most women, the rebound weight gains associated with diuretic use are usually temporary, lasting at most a month. Some women will return to their normal weight as quickly as five days after they stop taking diuretics. You may be able to offset some of this weight gain by adopting a low-sodium diet (see page 64) or switching to one of the potassium-sparing diuretics discussed above (ask your doctor for a prescription).

BREAST TENDERNESS (MASTALGIA)

Before resorting to drugs, you should first try wearing a good support bra and cutting back on caffeine. Some women also find vitamin E supplements and Evening Primrose Oil helpful (see pages 80 and 83 for more on these supplements).

If these measures don't sufficiently relieve breast tenderness, your physician may recommend that you take bromocriptine (Parlodel), a drug that blocks the release of the hormone prolactin from the pituitary gland.

Parlodel may cause some bothersome side effects, including nausea, vomiting, and dizziness. To minimize these side effects, it's best to start taking small doses of the drug at night before you go to bed, working your way up to larger doses after the first week.

Other medications your doctor may recommend for breast tenderness include birth control pills (although these sometimes worsen premenstrual symptoms—see page 115); *tamoxifen* (Nolvadex), an anti-estrogen typically used in the treatment of breast cancer; or *danazol* (Danocrine), a synthetic form of the male hormone testosterone (see also page 115).

PREMENSTRUAL CRAMPS, DIARRHEA, NAUSEA

A class of drugs known as *prostaglandin inhibitors*, such as *ibuprofen* (Motrin), *mefenamic acid* (Ponstel), and *naproxen* (Anaprox) are highly effective for symptoms of dysmenorrhea (painful periods) such as abdominal cramps, backache, headache, nausea, and vomiting, which often overlap with premenstrual symptoms. As their name implies, these drugs block the production of prostaglandins, which are suspected of playing a role in PMS. A handful of studies suggests that mefenamic acid and naproxen may also improve such PMS symptoms as fatigue, headaches, and mood swings. Prostaglandin inhibitors can also reduce the amount of bleeding during menstruation.

Your doctor may recommend that you take prostaglandin inhibitors a week before your period and continue to take them for the first day or two of menstruation. The drugs are safe and side effects are rare. Some women who are sensitive to aspirin may experience sensitivity to these drugs.

Many over-the-counter PMS formulas contain ibuprofen. If pain and discomfort are severe, your doctor may recommend that you take a stronger, prescription, medication such as Ponstel or Anaprox.

FATIGUE AND SLEEP DISTURBANCES

Some women may have no problem falling asleep at night but wake up in the middle of the night, unable to get back to sleep. Nighttime sleep disruptions can lead to daytime fatigue, irritability, and difficulty concentrating.

If you have problems sleeping, you should first try standard "sleep hygiene" measures. These include going to bed and getting up at the same time, using your bed only for sleep (and sex), and avoiding mentally or physically stimulating activities or substances (such as work, exercise, or caffeine-containing beverages) for several hours before bedtime. If you do wake up in the middle of the night, don't fight it; get up and do something relaxing, such as sewing, until you feel sleepy again.

If these measures don't work, your physician may recommend a tricyclic antidepressant, such as doxepin (Adapin, Sinequan), to be taken an hour or two before bedtime. You should avoid taking benzodiazepine "sleeping pills," as these are highly addictive.

MENSTRUAL MIGRAINE

If you suffer from predictable menstrual migraines, your physician may recommend that you take nonsteroidal anti-inflammatory drugs, such as naproxen, the week or two preceding your period as a preventive measure. If this type of therapy doesn't work, the antihypertensive drug *propranolol* (Inderal), or the antidepressant amitriptyline (Elavil, Etrafon) may be helpful in preventing migraines. Interestingly, estrogen (either oral estrogen or a single transdermal patch) may also be used to help prevent migraines. Low doses of estrogen beginning two or three days before the onset of menstruation and taken for seven days help stave off the drop in estrogen believed to trigger menstrual migraine. Sometimes estrogens are started just after ovulation. The drugs don't interfere with menstruation.

Danazol, a synthetic form of the male hormone testosterone, may also help prevent migraines when given in doses large enough to suppress ovulation. But this drug is associated with a number of bothersome side effects (see page 115).

WHAT ABOUT OVER-THE-COUNTER
PMS PREPARATIONS?

Pamprin, Midol, and other multisymptom menstrual preparations usually contain a pain reliever, such as ibuprofen or
acetaminophen, and one or more of the following "active
ingredients:"

Pyrilamine maleate, an antihistamine and sedative-hypnotic.
Preparations containing pyrilamine maleate may cause drowsiness, and you should avoid alcoholic beverages when taking
these medications, as alcohol may increase the sedative effects.

Pamabrom, a mild diuretic.

Caffeine, which has diuretic and analgesic properties.
Some over-the-counter menstrual products (usually "no-
drowsiness" formulas) contain up to 200 mg of caffeine (the
equivalent of two cups of coffee). But the substance is also a
potent stimulant, which can cause restlessness, sleep disturbances, and can trigger anxiety and panic attacks among
women with underlying anxiety or panic disorder. If you do
use an over-the-counter menstrual product, steer clear of those
containing caffeine.

Some women may find these preparations helpful for minor
premenstrual aches and pains, but for the most part, they are
ineffective in relieving mood swings and depression.

DEPRESSION, IRRITABILITY,
AND MOOD SWINGS

For women who suffer from irritability, depression, mood
swings, or other emotional symptoms, a number of options are
available. Oral micronized progesterone may be recommended
to help alleviate blue moods (see "What About Progesterone?"
below), although it has not been approved by the United States

Food and Drug Administration for this or any other use. The drug is usually started two or three days before symptoms are expected to begin.

If your major problem is depression, your physician may prescribe one of a number of antidepressant drugs, such as *fluoxetine* (Prozac) or *clomipramine* (Anafranil). If anxiety is a problem, anti-anxiety drugs, such as *buspirone* (BuSpar) or *alprazolam* (Xanax) may be prescribed.

Both antidepressant drugs and anti-anxiety drugs must be taken every day. Low doses of these psychotropic drugs usually work well for women with PMS, and side effects are uncommon.

WHAT ABOUT PROGESTERONE?

Although there's little conclusive evidence that it works, progesterone remains one of the most commonly used treatments for PMS. The treatment was first used in 1934, the same year the hormone was "discovered." The use of progesterone suppositories became more popular after British gynecologist Katharina Dalton published her book, *The Premenstrual Syndrome and Progesterone Therapy* (Year Book Medical Publishers, Chicago) in 1977 and again in 1984.

In theory, progesterone shows great promise in relieving many of the symptoms of PMS. Progesterone has diuretic properties, which could potentially relieve fluid retention and bloating. The hormone also relaxes smooth muscle and decreases the production of prostaglandins, which could theoretically reduce pain, nausea, vomiting, and diarrhea associated with PMS. Finally, the hormone has a sedative effect, which could help reduce premenstrual tension and anxiety.

In practice, however, there's little hard evidence that progesterone actually delivers the goods. In the 1980s, several small studies suggested that progesterone suppositories were no more effective than a placebo in relieving premenstrual depression and other symptoms. Proponents of progesterone therapy criticized these studies for their small size, short duration, and the use of low dosages of progesterone. So in 1990, Ellen Freeman, Ph.D., and colleagues at the University of Pennsylvania set out to settle the issue once and for all. They screened hundreds of women and recruited 168 with PMS to participate in their placebo-controlled, double-blind crossover study. During the study, the women first took a vaginal suppository—either placebo or 400 mg of progesterone—once in the morning from the sixteenth through the twenty-eighth day of one menstrual cycle. After one cycle on this treatment, the women taking a placebo were switched to the active drug, and the women taking progesterone were given a placebo for a menstrual cycle. During two more cycles of the study, the dosage was increased to two suppositories, or 800 mg of progesterone (400 mg in the morning and 400 mg at bedtime). Throughout the study the women kept daily symptom reports, which were used as the primary gauge of whether the treatment worked.

When the results were in, the progesterone suppository was found to be no better than the placebo in reducing the women's overall symptoms or any single symptom of PMS. The researchers concluded that "this method of progesterone therapy lacks sufficient effect to be clinically useful."

In spite of these findings, progesterone may still have a place in the treatment of PMS. Lorraine Dennerstein, M.D., and colleagues at the University of Melbourne in Australia found evidence that oral micronized progesterone capsules might be effective for certain symptoms. In a four-month study, the researchers gave twenty-three women either a placebo or 100 mg of oral micronized progesterone in the morning and another placebo or 200 mg of progesterone before bedtime for the last ten days of the menstrual cycle. At the end of the study, the progesterone capsules were found to be helpful in alleviating such symptoms as anxiety, depression, stress, swelling, hot flashes, and water retention.

The researchers speculated that oral progesterone may be broken down in the body (metabolized) differently than the progesterone in suppositories; oral progesterone is metabolized in the liver whereas progesterone in suppositories is absorbed directly into the bloodstream, bypassing the liver. These differences may account for oral progesterone's therapeutic effects. Of course, the study was small and lacks the statistical power of larger studies. Until larger studies are conducted, it's hard to say for certain whether oral micronized progesterone is truly beneficial.

If your physician *does* recommend that you try progesterone, you should know that the drug is considered quite safe. In more than sixty years of use, no serious complications have been reported among women using rectal or vaginal progesterone suppositories. But no drug is without side effects. One of the most common side effects associated with progesterone therapy is its sedative effect, which causes drowsiness, dizziness, and poor concentration in some women. (As we mentioned earlier, this sedative effect is also considered a therapeutic benefit of the drug.) Keep in mind, too, that some studies have found certain types of synthetic progestogens— notably medroxyprogesterone acetate (Provera), which is typically prescribed for postmenopausal women—to be associated with an increased incidence of mood swings and depression.

No studies have been conducted on any possible long-term side effects of vaginal or oral progesterone therapy.

SYNDROMAL THERAPY

Women with a variety of symptoms, including severe depression, irritability, or mood swings, may benefit from drugs that suppress ovulation.

BIRTH CONTROL PILLS

Premenstrual symptoms often clear up among women who take drugs that suppress ovulation, such as danazol and the newly discovered GnRH agonists (see below). So it seems only natural that birth control pills, which also suppress ovulation, would work, too. Studies have found, however, that birth control pills don't consistently help alleviate premenstrual symptoms. The use of oral contraceptives to treat PMS is complicated by the fact that combination birth control pills (those containing both estrogen and progestogen) have been associated with depression and other effects on mood.

If you suffer from PMS and need a reliable form of contraception, you may want to consider taking birth control pills for a few months to see if your symptoms subside. Some women actually do experience marked improvement in their symptoms when they start taking oral contraceptives. But for the majority of women who take them, symptoms remain unchanged or even worsen. If you decide to try oral contraceptives, use the newer low-dose pills.

DANAZOL (DANOCRINE)

Danazol is a synthetic form of the "male" hormone testosterone that has been used in the treatment of endometriosis and other gynecological problems. In fact, it was the coincidental improvement of PMS symptoms among women taking danazol for endometriosis that led researchers to investigate whether the drug might be useful in the treatment of PMS.

When taken daily, danazol suppresses the pituitary gland's release of follicle stimulating hormone and luteinizing hormone, in turn, decreasing the ovaries' secretion of estrogen and progesterone in the second half of the menstrual cycle.

D. H. Gilmore, M.D., a gynecologist in Glasgow, Scotland, found that doses of 400 mg per day relieved most premenstrual symptoms. But at these doses, the drug produces numerous unwanted side effects, including weight gain, nausea, giddiness, musculoskeletal pains, acne, excessive hair growth (including facial hair), a reduction in breast size, and deepening of the voice.

For this reason, researchers have investigated whether lower doses of danazol might also be effective. Several studies have reported improvements in premenstrual symptoms with just 100 mg of danazol twice a day—half the dose in Dr. Gilmore's study. In one study, twenty-four out of twenty-seven women reported improvements in their symptoms while taking 200 mg of danazol a day, compared with only six out of twenty-seven women taking a placebo. At this dosage, side effects were minor, including changes in menstruation (most women continued to bleed), nausea, and oily skin. Improvements in premenstrual symptoms come about because of the drug's ability to suppress ovulation.

GNRH AGONISTS
(LUPRON, SYNAREL)

Some of the most promising new drugs to come into use in recent years are GnRH agonists (brand name Lupron, Synarel).

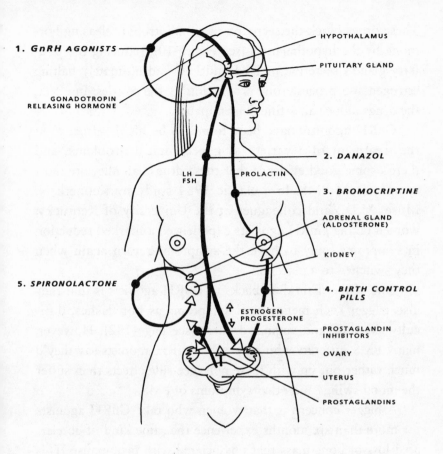

1. GnRH AGONISTS

GONADOTROPIN
RELEASING HORMONE

HYPOTHALAMUS

PITUITARY GLAND

2. DANAZOL

LH
FSH — PROLACTIN

3. BROMOCRIPTINE

ADRENAL GLAND
(ALDOSTERONE)

KIDNEY

5. SPIRONOLACTONE

**4. BIRTH CONTROL
PILLS**

ESTROGEN
PROGESTERONE

PROSTAGLANDIN
INHIBITORS

OVARY

UTERUS

PROSTAGLANDINS

FIGURE 10 Drugs used to treat PMS. (Drugs are in italics in the illustration.)
1. GnRH agonists block the production of gonadotropin releasing hormone by
the hypothalamus; this suppresses the release of follicle stimulating hormone
(FSH) and luteinizing hormone (LH) from the pituitary gland, inducing an artificial
menopause that usually clears up most premenstrual symptoms in severely
affected women. 2) Danazol suppresses the release of follicle stimulating
hormone and luteinizing hormone by the pituitary gland, preventing the monthly
release of an egg by the ovaries and the resulting fluctuations in estrogen and
progesterone that are thought to contribute to many premenstrual symptoms.
3) Bromocriptine stops the production of prolactin by the pituitary gland, which
helps relieve breast tenderness. 4) Like danazol, birth control pills also shut down
the pituitary gland's secretion of follicle stimulating hormone and luteinizing
hormone, suppressing ovulation. Oral contraceptives have not been found to be
terribly effective for the treatment of PMS. 5) The diuretic spironolactone
suppresses the secretion of aldosterone from the adrenal glands, which causes
the kidneys to release water. The drug is used to relieve premenstrual bloating
and water retention. 6) Prostaglandin inhibitors suppress the uterus' production
of prostaglandins, which cause premenstrual and menstrual cramps.

These drugs block the secretion of gonadotropin releasing hormone by the hypothalamus (see Figure 10), reducing the pituitary gland's secretion of FSH and LH, and ultimately halting estrogen and progesterone production by the ovaries. In effect, the drugs induce an artificial menopause.

GnRH agonists have been found to be highly effective in the treatment of a variety of gynecological problems, and there's some good evidence that these drugs can alleviate most symptoms of PMS. In a classic 1984 study by Kenneth N. Muse, M.D., and colleagues at the University of Kentucky, women taking GnRH agonists experienced a marked reduction in symptoms, only to have the symptoms return again when they switched to a placebo.

One of the main drawbacks to GnRH agonists is that they also trigger such menopausal symptoms as hot flashes, difficulty sleeping, and vaginal dryness (see page 132). However, many PMS sufferers who have used GnRH agonists say they'd much rather put up with these nuisance side effects than suffer the mood swings and other symptoms of PMS.

A bigger concern is that women who take GnRH agonists for more than six months experience the same kind of accelerated loss of bone mass that's associated with menopause. This could increase their risk of developing the bone-thinning disorder *osteoporosis* later in life. In addition, women who experience an early menopause are also known to be at an increased risk of developing heart disease, and there's a very real concern that women who take GnRH agonists for long periods of time would be at a greater risk, as well.

To counter the bone loss and potential risk of heart disease associated with long-term use of GnRH agonists, researchers are now investigating the use of standard postmenopausal hormone therapy (estrogen and progestogen) along with GnRH agonists in the treatment of PMS. Postmenopausal hormones have been proven to prevent osteoporosis and are believed to protect against heart disease in postmenopausal women who take them. But would adding estrogen and progestogen to this PMS treatment regimen simply cause premenstrual symptoms to return?

When low doses of estrogen and progestogen are given, this doesn't appear to be the case. In a 1991 study at the University of California-San Diego School of Medicine, J. F. Mortola, M.D., and colleagues treated eight women with GnRH agonists alone, and GnRH agonists together with estrogen and a progestogen. (Progestogen is given to help protect postmenopausal women from endometrial cancer.) To noone's surprise, symptoms improved 75 percent when the women took GnRH agonists alone. When GnRh agonists were given along with both estrogen and a progestogen were given together (estrogen throughout the entire cycle and progestogen just during the last half of the cycle), the women reported a 60 percent overall improvement in their symptoms.

Larger, long-term studies need to be conducted before scientists will know whether GnRH agonists together with standard postmenopausal hormone replacement therapy can improve premenstrual symptoms for long periods of time—and whether the drugs, individually and collectively, are safe. So far, the most serious long-term complications associated with GnRH agonists appear to be accelerated bone loss that could lead to osteoporosis, and an increased risk of heart disease, both of which can be offset by taking postmenopausal hormone therapy.

But how safe is postmenopausal hormone therapy? From what scientists know so far, postmenopausal hormones are surprisingly safe, and for most women, the benefits of these drugs far outweigh the risks. Here's how things stand now:

ENDOMETRIAL CANCER

Postmenopausal women who have not had a hysterectomy (surgical removal of the uterus) and who take estrogen alone are at an increased risk of developing endometrial cancer. This is because estrogen alone overstimulates the uterine lining, causing an overgrowth of cells that in a small number of women—about four in one thousand—could develop into cancer. But when a progestogen is given along with the estrogen, the combination actually *protects against endometrial cancer. This is why you must take a progestogen along with an estrogen if you have not had a hysterectomy.*

HEART DISEASE

Because the hormones in birth control pills have been associated with an increased risk of cardiovascular disease, scientists worried that postmenopausal estrogens might also raise a woman's risk of heart disease. It now appears that postmenopausal estrogens—which are given in much lower doses than birth control pills, and have a different chemical make-up than the estrogens in oral contraceptives—actually protect against heart disease. Indeed, numerous population studies have shown that *women who take postmenopausal estrogens are half as likely to suffer a heart attack as those who don't take estrogens.* It's still not certain what effect, if any, added progestogens will have on a woman's heart disease risk, however. That's still under investigation.

BREAST CANCER

One of the unresolved safety issues associated with postmenopausal estrogens is the possibility that long-term use of these drugs may increase a woman's risk of developing breast cancer. This fear was fueled by a 1989 Swedish study involving more than 23,000 post-menopausal women ages thirty-five and older. While the study showed that women using a combination of estrogen and progestogen experienced overall only about 10 percent more breast cancers than expected, women in the study who took estrogen for more than nine years had a much higher than expected incidence of breast cancer. Most studies, however, have shown only a slightly increased risk of breast cancer (about 30 percent) among women who take postmenopausal estrogen for 15 years or longer. No studies have shown an increase in deaths from breast cancer among estrogen users, and some have actually shown an increase in the cure rate of breast cancer among women taking postmenopausal hormones!

Keep in mind that the breast cancer question may be more relevant for postmenopausal women than for premenopausal women taking GnRH agonists. The reason: when post-menopausal women take estrogen, they're artificially extending the number of years they are exposed to estrogen, and there's some concern that by doing so, these women may increase their risk of developing breast cancer. On the other hand, pre-menopausal women taking estrogen add-back therapy along with GnRH agonists are simply replacing the estrogen their bodies normally would be producing anyway.

On the other hand, if you have a family history of breast cancer and you take estrogen, your risk of developing breast cancer is about double that of women who don't take estrogen. For this reason, many women whose mothers or sisters have been diagnosed with breast cancer are often advised *not* to take estrogen.

One way to help offset any potential increased risk of breast cancer is to examine your breasts every month using breast self-examination (ask your doctor to show you how), and have your physician or another health care professional examine your breasts at least once a year. If you are over age forty and take postmenopausal estrogens, you should have a mammogram every two to three years, as well.

GnRH agonists, together with postmenopausal hormone therapy, are one of the most promising, safe, and effective treatments for PMS to come along. But because some questions about the safety and efficacy of these drugs remain unanswered, only women with severe PMS that seriously interferes with their lives are candidates for this type of drug therapy. Ultimately, the combination of GnRH agonists and postmenopausal hormone therapy may prove to be an ideal long-term therapy for women with the most severe cases of PMS. For now, short-term use of this combination drug therapy may be used as a kind of litmus test to determine whether women with severe PMS would benefit from having their ovaries surgically removed, which, right now, is the only permanent "cure" for PMS. (For more on the surgical treatment of PMS, see Chapter 7.)

If your physician recommends that you try GnRH agonists, make sure you fully understand the benefits and risks of these medications before taking them, and the importance of taking postmenopausal hormone therapy along with them.

CHAPTER 7

CAN A HYSTERECTOMY CURE PMS?

If you have severe PMS that doesn't seem to respond to the usual therapeutic measures, you may have found yourself thinking on more than one occasion, "Maybe I should just have a hysterectomy and be done with it."

Surgery is such a drastic measure that many physicians don't even consider it to be a viable option for women with PMS. In fact, surgery *is* an option for women with PMS. But it's expensive, potentially risky, and irreversible. For these reasons, it should be considered only as a last resort, when all other therapeutic measures have failed. And it should be considered only by women with the most severe, debilitating cases of PMS who have completed their families.

Only you can determine whether your symptoms are severe enough to warrant such a radical treatment. Before you decide, you owe it to yourself to learn as much as you can about the operation, its potential short- and long-term complications, and how you can deal with them. Here are some considerations to keep in mind.

WHAT IS A HYSTERECTOMY?

Although hysterectomy is the second most commonly performed surgical procedure in the United States (cesarean sections top the list), many women are confused about just what a hysterectomy is. In simplest terms, a hysterectomy is an operation in which a woman's uterus is removed. If you have a *simple hysterectomy, your ovaries are left intact.* If you have this operation before you experience a natural menopause, your ovaries will continue to function, secreting the hormones estrogen and progesterone and releasing an egg once a month, just as they did before your operation—you just won't have a monthly menstrual period to remind you. Contrary to popular belief, a total hysterectomy does not mean that the ovaries are removed along with the uterus. Rather, this term refers to the surgical removal of the uterus and cervix. The ovaries are unaffected.

When both of the woman's ovaries are removed along with her uterus and fallopian tubes—what many women think of as a total hysterectomy—the operation is known as a *hysterectomy with bilateral salpingo-oophorectomy.* (To simplify matters, we will refer to this procedure as a *hysterectomy and ovariectomy*, or simply *ovariectomy*.) If you have this type of surgery before menopause, you will suddenly cease producing the hormones estrogen and progesterone and will undergo an instantaneous or "surgical" menopause, complete with hot flashes, vaginal dryness, and a host of other menopause-related health problems.

HYSTERECTOMY OR OVARIECTOMY FOR PMS?

As you may have already surmised, a hysterectomy alone generally will not cure PMS, since your ovaries remain intact and continue to function. However, a few small studies have demonstrated that some women who undergo a simple hysterectomy experience a reduction in the number and severity of their symptoms. It's possible that hysterectomy may have worked in these cases by removing a major source of certain prostaglandins—the uterus. (Remember, prostaglandins have been implicated as a possible cause of some premenstrual symptoms.) But for the most part, the ability of simple hysterectomy to alleviate premenstrual symptoms is so-so, and most experts agree that surgical removal of the uterus is too radical a treatment to consider if the results are lukewarm, at best.

Having just one ovary removed isn't an effective surgical treatment for PMS, either, as the other will compensate for the loss by ovulating every month and producing the estrogen and progesterone necessary to regulate your menstrual cycle. *The only effective surgical treatment for PMS is to have both ovaries removed along with your uterus.*

How effective is this type of surgery? Obviously, it's impossible to compare this treatment with a placebo, since subjecting women to major surgery and removing the ovaries of some women but not others without telling them would be considered medically unethical. But the results of two small studies published in 1990, both involving women with severe PMS, are impressive. Gynecologist P. Casson, M.D., and colleagues at Queen's University in Ontario, Canada, performed surgery on 14 women with PMS who found no other relief from their debilitating symptoms. All of the women reported a dramatic improvement in their everyday mood, their overall sense of well-being, and the quality of their lives after having their ovaries removed. In a similar study, this one at the University of Western Ontario in Canada, Robert F. Casper, M.D., and Margaret T. Hearn, Ph.D., surgically treated 14 women whose PMS symptoms were so severe that their home and work lives were disrupted three weeks out of every month. After the surgery, the women participating in the study reported that their lives had turned around and that they were completely satisfied with the results of the surgery.

WEIGHING THE RISKS

If having your ovaries removed is so effective in relieving the symptoms of PMS, why don't all women with PMS have surgery? Because this operation—like any type of surgery—is not without risks. These include risks associated with the operation itself and—perhaps more importantly—several potentially serious long-term effects on your health. *Indeed, the two most serious long-term health risks associated with ovariectomy—an increased risk of heart disease and osteoporosis—are greatest for premenopausal women like yourself.* Fortunately, most of these complications—including many of the long-term health risks—can be managed. Here's a closer look at some of the major risks associated with surgical removal of the ovaries.

Short-Term Risks

Thanks to advances in surgical procedures, anesthetics, and antibiotics, hysterectomy and ovariectomy are among the safest operations performed today. But as we mentioned earlier, no surgery is without risks. Some of the short-term risks associated with ovariectomy are anesthesia-related complications, possible hemorrhage (uncontrolled bleeding) and subsequent reactions to blood transfusions, injury to adjacent organs, such as the bowel or urinary tract, and postoperative infection. In addition, your uterus helps support other organs in the pelvic cavity, such as your vagina and bladder, and changes in your anatomy after having a hysterectomy can sometimes result in prolapse, or "sagging" of other organs, which can only be corrected with further surgery.

Keep in mind that while deaths associated with the operation itself are extremely rare, they do occasionally occur. Estimates range from 4.1 to 85.1 per 10,000 women, depending on which study you look at. At greatest risk are women who have pregnancy-related hysterectomies, women who have cancer-related hysterectomies and women over age sixty-five.

Menopausal Symptoms

Unlike women who go through a natural menopause and experience a gradual reduction in estrogen and progesterone over several years' time, the body's production of these hormones comes to a screeching halt in premenopausal women who have their ovaries removed. For this reason, surgically menopausal women often experience more and more severe symptoms of menopause, such as hot flashes, sleep disruptions, and vaginal dryness. Usually, these problems can be comfortably managed by taking estrogen.

Depression and Sexual Problems

A minority of women who have their uterus removed may be more prone to suffer from depression, anxiety, and sexual problems after surgery—what has been labeled *posthysterectomy syndrome*. There's no clear explanation for why this might occur. Scientists have speculated that depression could stem from the unique significance of the uterus and its function to women. Some experts suggest that the removal of this child-bearing organ, which so influences a woman's bodily processes and reflects her feminine nature, can have a profound psychological effect. Right now, however, there's no good evidence to back up these theories.

Preliminary research suggests that women at greatest risk of suffering posthysterectomy syndrome are those who have their ovaries removed along with the uterus (which of course would include any woman undergoing a hysterectomy and ovariectomy in hopes of curing PMS), women who had sexual problems prior to surgery, and women who see their attractiveness and femininity tied up in their reproductive ability. Preoperative counseling may be helpful in preventing some of the postoperative emotional turmoil. You should note, too, that most healthy women adjust without feeling that their worth as women has been compromised.

While there appears to be no psychological reason for your sexual appetite or responsiveness to change after you've had a hysterectomy, some women do report a postoperative decline in sexual responsiveness. This could be because the uterus plays a peripheral role in orgasms. Often, women who develop sexual problems after surgery can be helped by a reputable counselor or sex therapist.

Heart Disease

It is becoming increasingly clear that estrogen provides women with a kind of built-in biological protection against heart disease through their childbearing years. But this immunity runs out after menopause (both natural and surgically induced), when a woman's risk of heart disease rises dramatically. Indeed, heart disease is the leading cause of death among women ages forty and over.

One reason for the rise in a woman's heart disease risk after menopause may be partly related to the effects of estrogen on cholesterol, a fatty substance circulating in the bloodstream. High blood levels of cholesterol are associated with *atherosclerosis*, or progressive narrowing of the arteries that can predispose you to a heart attack or stroke. The drop in estrogen after menopause is linked with an increase in total blood cholesterol and the "bad" LDL cholesterol, believed to increase your risk of heart disease, as well as a reduction in the "good" HDL cholesterol, thought to protect against heart disease. Estrogen's effects on blood cholesterol may not be the only way in which the hormone provides protection from heart disease; estrogen may work in other ways, as well.

Women who have their ovaries removed before experiencing a natural menopause lose this protection against heart disease much sooner than women who don't have the operation. (The average age of women who experience a natural menopause is fifty-one.) As a result, surgically menopausal women are at a much greater risk of developing heart disease than their naturally menopausal counterparts. In fact, women who undergo an ovariectomy before age thirty-five *are seven times more likely to develop coronary heart disease* than women who don't have this operation.

If you have an ovariectomy, one important way to protect yourself against this increased risk of heart disease is to take estrogen. Indeed, numerous studies have shown that *postmenopausal women who take estrogen are roughly half as likely to suffer a heart attack as women who don't take hormones.*

Osteoporosis

Estrogen has a protective effect on your bones as well as your heart. After menopause, the gradual loss of bone mass associated with normal aging occurs at a more rapid clip. If you have a low bone mass to begin with, or if you continue to lose bone mass rapidly for many years, your bones may weaken to the point that debilitating fractures (typically of the spine, wrist, or hip) may occur with even the slightest provocation—a serious condition known as *osteoporosis*.

Osteoporosis can be painful, crippling, and sometimes fatal. (Osteoporosis is the twelfth leading cause of death among women today.) And because surgically menopausal women lose the protective effects of estrogen on their bones years earlier than naturally menopausal women, they are at a much greater risk of developing osteoporosis later in life. Indeed, from 25 to 50 percent of women who have had both ovaries removed prior to a natural menopause will develop osteoporosis at a relatively early age if they do not take post-menopausal estrogens.

There's no cure for osteoporosis, but it can be prevented. And one of the best ounces of prevention for surgically menopausal women is to take postmenopausal estrogens. Estrogen users have about half the number of hip fractures as nonusers. And in 1980, Robert Lindsey, M.D., of Columbia University's College of Physicians and Surgeons in New York documented a 90 percent drop in spinal deformities (such as loss of height and the Dowager's hump) among surgically menopausal women who took estrogen for at least ten years.

Getting plenty of weight-bearing exercise (such as walking or jogging) and getting enough calcium from your diet can help reduce your risk, too. But you should be aware that loading up on calcium supplements simply isn't enough to slow bone loss and help offset the risk of osteoporosis associated with a surgical menopause. *You really should take estrogen, too.*

HORMONE THERAPY: WEIGHING THE RISKS

As you can see, postmenopausal hormone therapy plays a critical role in preventing most of the long-term health risks associated with ovariectomy, and *if you choose to have an ovariectomy for the treatment of PMS, you really should commit yourself to taking estrogen for many years after your surgery to offset these potentially serious long-term health threats.* But as with all drugs, postmenopausal estrogens have risks, too. And since estrogen therapy is an integral part of the ultimate success of your surgery, you should know the facts about this drug, as well.

You have probably heard or read by now that estrogen increases a woman's risk of endometrial cancer (cancer of the uterine lining). Fortunately, this is one risk you *won't* have to worry about if you are taking estrogen after a hysterectomy and ovariectomy, the risk is increased only for women with an intact uterus. (Doctors rarely remove a woman's ovaries without also removing her uterus. Moreover, women with an intact uterus can safely take estrogen without having to worry about endometrial cancer provided they also take a progestogen along with estrogen; this combination has actually been found to protect against endometrial cancer!)

Breast cancer is another issue—and a sticky one, too. Because certain types of breast cancer are fueled by the hormone estrogen, and because a woman's age at menarche (start of menstruation), age at first birth, and age at menopause appear to affect her subsequent chances of getting breast cancer, the hormones used to treat postmenopausal women have come under close scrutiny. Most current evidence suggests that postmenopausal estrogens either have no effect on your risk of breast cancer or that the hormones cause only a slightly elevated risk when used for more than fifteen years, or when taken in relatively high doses. Moreover, no studies have shown an increase in deaths from breast cancer among estrogen users, and some have actually shown an increase in the cure rate of breast cancer among women taking postmenopausal estrogens. Moreover, the breast cancer question may *not* be relevant to premenopausal women who have their ovaries removed, since these women would normally be producing estrogen anyway—at least until age fifty-one, the average age of menopause.

If you have a family history of breast cancer, however, you should carefully discuss with your doctor the pros and cons of taking postmenopausal estrogens after an ovariectomy. Several studies have shown that when postmenopausal women with a family history of breast cancer take estrogen, their risk of developing breast cancer is double that of women who don't take estrogen. On the other hand, certain estrogen preparations (those containing only the hormone estradiol, such as Estrace) are easily monitored in the bloodstream and sometimes may be safely used by women with a family history of breast cancer.

Interestingly, removal of a woman's ovaries before age forty is associated with a lifelong reduction in breast cancer risk of about 50 percent. But again, this protection must be weighed against the increased risk of osteoporosis and heart disease among surgically menopausal women who don't take estrogen.

Another concern you may have is whether taking post-menopausal estrogens will trigger PMS-like symptoms in you—again. After all, studies have shown that postmenopausal women who take estrogen along with progestogen *do* sometimes experience PMS-like symptoms. These mood swings and depression have been linked to the progestogen the women take, not the estrogen. You won't have to take progestogen, so this shouldn't be a problem.

WILL OVARIECTOMY WORK FOR YOU?

Before you and your physician make a final decision to have surgery, your doctor will probably insist that you take either danazol or GnRH agonists together with estrogen and progestogen add-back therapy for several months. (If your doctor doesn't insist, *you* should.) As you may recall, these drugs induce an artificial menopause (see page 118) and serve as an ideal screening and diagnostic test for women who are considering surgery for the treatment of PMS. In fact, GnRH agonists may soon replace surgery altogether as a long-term treatment for women with severe PMS.

If your symptoms don't abate while you are taking these drugs, surgery probably won't be of much help to you, either. In fact, the failure of these drugs to alleviate your symptoms may strongly suggest that your primary problem isn't PMS. On the other hand, if you notice a significant improvement in your symptoms, you may want to consider seriously having surgery—at least until GnRH agonists are proven to be safe and effective for the long-term treatment of women with PMS. Using GnRH agonists along with estrogen add-back therapy has another advantage: it allows you to see how you will respond to the estrogen therapy you'll need to stave off the long-term health risks associated with ovariectomy.

Because an ovariectomy is irreversible, you should carefully think through the pros and cons of this type of therapy before making a decision. It helps to learn as much as you can about the operation itself. Talk to your doctor and to other women who have had their ovaries removed—even if they've had the operation for a condition other than PMS. These women can give you a better idea of what to expect after surgery. If you *do* opt for surgery, you should plan on a four- to seven-day hospital stay and a six- to eight-week recovery time, so you will have to make appropriate arrangements with your employer and your family for time off. Since you will be advised not to drive a car or lift heavy objects (or children) for four to six weeks after the operation, *you will need help*, particularly during the first week or two after you are discharged from the hospital. You can also expect to experience a considerable amount of pain while you are in the hospital and continued discomfort for several weeks after your operation. Your doctor will prescribe pain medication to help keep you comfortable. Even so, you will probably feel some discomfort for a while.

Obviously, you shouldn't even think about having an ovariectomy if you have not yet completed your family or if you have any doubts whatsoever about whether you might want children some time in the future. Once you have this operation, you won't be able to change your mind later on.

If you do choose to have an ovariectomy, you will have to make a firm commitment to take extra good care of yourself in the years to come to help fend off the long-term health risks of heart disease and osteoporosis. As we mentioned before, taking estrogen is one of the best ways to protect yourself from these long-term complications. But eating right and exercising regularly are equally important.

Finally, you'll have to make sure your physician is willing to perform the operation. Many doctors won't even consider performing surgery if your only reason for having an ovariectomy is relief of PMS. Some are more willing if you also have another compelling reason to have a hysterectomy—extremely painful periods, for instance, heavy bleeding, a (benign) fibroid tumor of the uterus, or painful endometriosis. If you and your doctor have a philosophical disagreement and you are convinced that surgery is right for you, you should first seek a second opinion—and perhaps even a third. Also, don't forget to ask your insurance carrier whether it will cover the operation.

If you can honestly say that your symptoms are troublesome enough to justify the time, pain, expense, and potential long-term health risks involved in this type of surgery, then perhaps an ovariectomy is the right option for you.

CHAPTER 8

LEARNING TO LIVE WITH PMS

As you know, there's no cure for PMS, but you can learn to cope with the symptoms. Here's how three women managed.

JANET'S STORY

From the time she was a teenager, Janet recalls being a moody person. "I just thought it was part of my personality," says the forty-three-year-old technical editor. She had even seen a psychiatrist as a young adult and was told she had a "mood disorder."

As she got older, Janet's mood swings intensified. So did the fights she had with her husband. "I'd threaten to break up our marriage," she recalls. "He never knew where he stood with me. He was a dedicated, loyal husband and it was difficult for him to be confronted like this."

But over the years, Janet's husband began to notice something she hadn't. The fights seemed to occur on a regular basis, shortly before her monthly menstrual period. Finally, he confronted her: "Don't you realize that you're getting your period and your moods are cyclical?" he told her one morning when she was feeling particularly down. She looked hard at herself in the mirror that day and thought, "Maybe he's right."

Shortly afterward, Janet spotted an ad in the newspaper announcing the formation of a support group for women with

PMS. The meeting was free, so Janet decided she had nothing to lose. When she attended the meeting, she found that she was not alone, that other women experienced symptoms and problems similar to hers. "It was such a relief to see other women going through the same thing I was," she says. Janet also learned that there was a great deal that could be done to control her symptoms, including the mood swings and irritability that were taxing her marriage. "I knew I had to do something to get rid of this," recalls Janet, who describes herself as a take-charge, self-disciplined person. So the following week, Janet made an appointment with the gynecologist at the women's health clinic that had sponsored the support group.

After undergoing a physical examination, the first thing Janet was advised to do was to chart her symptoms. Each day before she went to bed, she'd rank the intensity of her worst symptoms—irritability, anger, mood swings, breast tenderness, and food cravings. After two months, she saw clearly what her husband had suspected: her symptoms were, in fact, occurring cyclically. And while her PMS wasn't debilitating, it had become a considerable source of marital stress. "The biggest problem I had was not with my co-workers or friends, but with the person closest to me—my husband," she recalls. "We had countless unnecessary fights. I knew that he loved me, but when I was getting my period, I could be unkind and thoughtless, knowing that he would still have to love me because we were married."

Because her symptoms weren't severe and because she preferred not to take medication, Janet decided to try some of the self-help measures recommended by the clinic. Janet already exercised regularly, and she was encouraged to keep it up. She also met with the clinic's registered dietitian who, after conducting a nutritional analysis of Janet's diet, advised her to cut back on her caffeine, salt, and sugar intake during the week or two before her period to help reduce breast tenderness and swelling.

One of the most helpful and therapeutic measures Janet took was simply to chart her symptoms. Keeping a record of her symptoms helped make Janet more aware of what was happening to her. "Now when I see on the calendar that my period is approaching, I know to be more gentle to myself and others."

MARYANN'S STORY

Maryann's problems didn't begin until after the birth of her third child. She had had a tubal ligation (a form of contraception in which the Fallopian tubes are blocked), and while she and her husband (a physician) couldn't find a connection between the surgical procedure and PMS in the medical literature, she is convinced that the operation in some way contributed to her problems. "I never had a problem before that time," she recalls. "And although there was nothing in the medical literature about tubal ligations and PMS, I have spoken with a lot of other women who said that after they had a tubal ligation, their PMS was definitely worse."

A year and a half later, Maryann's symptoms—weight gain, bloating, and heavy periods, along with premenstrual irritability and depression—were bad enough that she made an appointment with her gynecologist. After a quick physical examination, the doctor recommended that Maryann see a counselor. "But I knew it was more than that," recalls Maryann.

In the meantime, Maryann's irritability and depression began to take its toll on her and her family. "Even fixing dinner or going to the store or taking care of my kids was a real challenge. I felt at times as though I couldn't think straight, as though my whole personality was changing. I don't normally yell, but when I was premenstrual, I found myself constantly yelling at my kids. Then I started retreating into my room so I wouldn't yell at the kids anymore. Fortunately, I had a very understanding husband. He'd come in and help with the children, cook dinner, or do the dishes. I don't know what I would have done without him."

When her symptoms failed to improve, Maryann sought the help of an endocrinologist (hormone specialist) at a nearby teaching hospital. The doctor recommended that she start taking progesterone in September of 1989. But by January 1990, Maryann wasn't any better. That month, she had a severe and prolonged period lasting ten days. An endometrial biopsy (in which the doctor removes a small sample of the uterine lining) ruled out endometrial cancer, but also failed to determine the cause of the bleeding.

Six months later, because the bleeding had become a chronic problem, Maryann's doctor recommended that she have a hysterectomy and ovariectomy. "At that time, I was either having PMS or fifteen-day periods, so I never had a good day."

Maryann's depression didn't improve after the operation— an indication that she may have been experiencing an underlying depression all along. On the advice of her physician, Maryann sought the help of a counselor and, when it became obvious that she needed antidepressant drugs, a psychiatrist. "The counseling was enormously helpful," says Maryann. "I was the one who tried to keep the peace in the family, who tried to make my husband and kids happy. And I had a tendency to hold things in. The therapist helped me voice legitimate complaints that I had with my husband."

"The counselor also helped me to say 'no' when people asked me to help with one thing or another. So many people think, 'Oh, you're a stay-at-home mom; you can help out with school or volunteer at church.' The therapist helped me learn how to say, 'No I'm not going to get involved in extracurricular activities right now. I need to take care of myself.' As a result," says Maryann, "I'm starting to have good days. I think I'm finally on the upswing."

CECILIA'S STORY

It wasn't until Cecilia got pregnant with her first child at age thirty-four that she realized how much her premenstrual symptoms affected her. "After the nausea and fatigue of the first three months of pregnancy cleared up, I felt better than I had in my entire adult life," she says.

After the baby was born, Cecilia's premenstrual symptoms returned and she never again felt quite as good as she did during her pregnancy. Her symptoms were vague—bloating, confusion, memory lapses, and clumsiness—and because her son was often up all night with ear problems, she tended to chalk up many of her symptoms to a lack of sleep.

Within a year after the baby was born, Cecilia had moved to a different town and began searching for a new doctor. The first recommended that she drink a few cups of coffee to ease her premenstrual bloating, since caffeine is a diuretic. She knew caffeine could exacerbate premenstrual symptoms, so she decided instead to go to another doctor.

Cecilia's new gynecologist gave her a prescription for progesterone and another for the anti-anxiety medication Xanax. The drugs seemed to help initially, but during the next year or so, her symptoms worsened, in spite of an increase in medication. Then her symptoms became so debilitating that she simply couldn't function anymore. "One month, I sat down to pay the bills and my mind was in such a fog that I sent the water bill to the electric company, and I forgot to sign or date most of the checks. Within a few days, the checks all started coming back, and it took a month to straighten out the mess." The following month, as Cecilia was driving around town running errands, she got lost—even though she knew her way around town quite well. "I simply could not figure out how to get home," she recalls. She kept dropping things at work, too. Then one day, while she was taking the groceries out of the car, "I started screaming at my little boy because he wouldn't help me carry the groceries into the house, even though he was too little to help." That incident, says Cecilia, was the last straw. She called her gynecologist that day and together, they decided that she should see a specialist in PMS. They decided on Dr. Rapkin because she was the closest.

As a patient of Dr. Rapkin, Cecilia agreed to participate in a study involving a new treatment regimen—the GnRH agonist Lupron along with hormone replacement therapy. "By the end of the third month, I started feeling great. My thoughts cleared up, my skin cleared up, I really felt wonderful."

Because Cecilia did so well while taking Lupron, she is now trying to decide whether to have her ovaries surgically removed. "I'm still not sure whether I'm ready for that," she adds.

CHAPTER 9

A BETTER TOMORROW

Congratulations! By learning about the possible causes of PMS and the various treatment options available to you, you've just taken the first step in gaining control over your symptoms and, to a certain extent, your life.

Now take the next step. Begin charting your symptoms. Over the next several months, you'll begin to see that your symptoms do follow a fairly predictable pattern. You may even begin to recognize some of the subtle early warning signs your body sends you; perhaps you'll notice a slight puffiness around the nipples of your breasts a day or two before the pain sets in. Or you may find that the music on the radio, which normally sounds pleasant to you, suddenly seems loud and irritating. What a relief it will be for you to realize that you're not "losing it" or spiraling out of control, you're just getting your period.

Scientists are constantly increasing their understanding about the causes of PMS; every day brings them closer to developing new and more effective treatment options. Still, for the moment, there's no cure for PMS, and right now, your goal is to learn how to manage your symptoms so they don't overwhelm you. If you have mild to moderate symptoms, you may be able to manage quite well by exercising regularly and cutting back on sodium in your diet the week or two before your period. If you have severe, debilitating symptoms, you will most definitely need the help of your physician *and* a professional counselor or therapist. And while it may take several months before you find the treatment approach that's right for you, try to be patient.

Above all, during the week before your period, be good to yourself. Your symptoms are your body's way of telling you to take it easy. Listen to your body. If you're tired and your schedule permits, indulge in a nap. If you feel you need some time to yourself, tell your family and friends how you feel and set aside some quiet time—your lunch hour, perhaps, or a half-hour or so after dinner—to read a favorite book or engage in another enjoyable activity. If you feel weepy, sometimes it's better just to have a good cry and get it out of your system than to hold it in and prolong your misery—no apologies needed. A good way to handle negative feelings is to set a time limit for them and stick to it. Tell yourself, "I'm going to let myself feel down and depressed for the next hour. Then I'm not going to be depressed anymore." You'd be surprised at how well this approach works.

Most women who seek treatment for PMS eventually will see a noticeable improvement in their symptoms. You are bound to feel better, too. And with a positive, take-charge attitude, tomorrow will be a better day.

APPENDIX

American College of Obstetricians and Gynecologists
Resource Center
409 12th Street SW
Washington, DC 20024

The College provides free brochures on a wide range of women's health topics, including premenstrual syndrome, endometriosis, hysterectomy, and postmenopausal hormone therapy. Send a self-addressed, stamped business envelope along with your request for information.

American Dietetic Association
National Center for Nutrition and Dietetics
216 West Jackson Blvd, Suite 800
Chicago, IL 60606-6995

If you wish to take a nutritional approach to PMS, you may want to contact this professional organization, which can provide you with a list of registered dietitians in your area. Although the R.D.s don't necessarily specialize in nutritional approaches to the treatment of PMS, most can perform a nutritional analysis and counsel you on how you can improve your eating habits, providing practical advice on cutting back on sodium, sugar, and fat in your diet. In addition to providing referrals to registered dietitians in your area, the organization also publishes a variety of materials on nutrition and good eating habits. Write for referrals and for a publication list.

National Institute of Child Health and Human Development
PO Box 29111
Washington, DC 20040

This branch of the National Institutes of Health supports research in the reproductive sciences and publishes a free, informative fact sheet entitled *Dysmenorrhea and Premenstrual Syndrome*. For a copy of the fact sheet, write to the NICHHD at the address above.

National Women's Health Network
1325 G Street NW
Washington, DC 20005

This nonprofit information service offers information packets on PMS and a number of other women's health topics. Smaller information packets (five to ten pages) are free with a written request; larger packets (forty to fifty pages) cost $5.00. The Network can also provide you with a list of women's health clinics in your area that may or may not specialize in the treatment of PMS. (The organization does not have the resources to provide individual physician referrals.) For more information, write to the National Women's Health Network at the above address.

GLOSSARY

Aldosterone: a hormone secreted by the adrenal glands that helps regulate the body's salt and water balance.

Amines: brain chemicals, including serotonin, tyramine and norepinephrine, that play a role in nerve impulse transmission. Some amines (histamine and serotonin) cause dilation of blood vessels and are believed to play a role in triggering migraine headaches.

Angiotensin: a chemical in the blood that causes blood vessels to constrict and that stimulates the release of *aldosterone* from the adrenal glands, helping to maintain the body's sodium and fluid balance.

Arachidonic acid: a fatty acid commonly found in animal fats (meat and dairy products) that the body uses to help make prostaglandins.

Basal body temperature: the temperature of the body taken in the morning before rising or moving about or eating or drinking anything. A slight rise in the basal body temperature can be used to predict a woman's time of ovulation.

Beta-endorphins: see *endorphins*.

Bromocriptine (Parlodel): a drug that blocks the pituitary gland's production of prolactin. The drug is sometimes prescribed to relieve premenstrual breast pain.

Caffeine: a food additive and "active ingredient" in hundreds of foods, beverages, and over-the-counter and prescription medications. Caffeine has diuretic and analgesic properties and is a potent central nervous system stimulant.

Calcium: a mineral found in certain foods (particularly milk and dairy products) and in the body, where it is used to harden teeth and bones, and for muscle contraction, blood clotting, and nerve impulse transmission. Its role in triggering or relieving premenstrual symptoms is not clear.

Circadian rhythms: a term used to describe the body's biological "clock" or rhythms, such as the natural sleep-wake cycle in a 24-hour period. Desynchronization of the body's biological clock can affect biological, mental, and behavioral functions.

Complex carbohydrates: starchy foods, such as potatoes, rice, pasta, bulgar, couscous, millet, corn, peas and beans, as well as fruits and vegetables. These foods are high in dietary fiber and vitamins and low in calories and fat.

Corpus luteum: the empty egg sac that produces the hormone progesterone after ovulation.

Cushing's syndrome: a disorder resulting from excessive production of the hormone cortisol by the adrenal glands, or by prolonged administration of certain drugs. Symptoms include mental or emotional disturbances, high blood pressure, weight gain, and abnormal growth of facial and body hair.

Danazol (Danocrine): a synthetic form of the male hormone testosterone. When given in high enough doses, danazol suppresses ovulation. The drug has been used in the treatment of endometriosis and has also been used to treat women with severe PMS.

Depression: an emotional state marked by feelings of sadness, discouragement and hopelessness, often accompanied by reduced activity, unresponsiveness, apathy and sleep disturbances. There are two types: major depression (also known as unipolar depression), and manic-depressive illness (also known as bipolar depression), characterized by cycles of depression and elation or mania. Both types are believed to have biochemical, genetic, and environmental roots. Treatment may include psychotherapy, antidepressant drugs, or both. Electroshock therapy is sometimes used to treat people with manic-depressive illness.

Diuretics: drugs that increase the kidneys' excretion of salt and water. There are several kinds, each of which affects a different part of the kidney: loop and thiazide diuretics are generally prescribed for the treatment of high blood pressure and congestive heart failure. The milder potassium-sparing diuretics, so named because they help the body retain potassium, are usually prescribed for premenstrual fluid retention. Over-the-counter diuretics; the mildest of all, contain the active ingredients pamabrom or ammonium-chloride.

Dopamine: one of several neurotransmitters in the brain that allows nerve cells to communicate with one another. Low levels of dopamine are associated with depression.

Dysmenorrhea: painful periods characterized by cramps, nausea, vomiting, and other discomforts that begin just before or with the onset of menstruation. Women with dysmenorrhea often complain of premenstrual symptoms, as well. Prostaglandin-inhibitors are the initial treatment of choice for these symptoms.

Edema: fluid retention in the body's tissues that may cause puffiness, bloating, breast tenderness, and weight gain.

Endometriosis: a condition in which parts of the uterine lining (endometrium) grow outside of the uterus, causing pelvic pain, painful periods, pain during intercourse, and pain with defecation. The condition can sometimes lead to infertility. For reasons that aren't clear, many women with endometriosis also suffer from premenstrual syndrome.

Endometrium: the inner mucus layer of the uterus that thickens in preparation for pregnancy each month under the influence of the hormones estrogen and progesterone and is shed if pregnancy doesn't occur.

Endorphins: naturally occurring chemicals in the brain believed to be involved in reducing or eliminating pain and enhancing pleasure. Exercise is believed to raise levels of endorphins; some researchers theorize that premenstrual symptoms may actually be withdrawal symptoms resulting from a drop in endorphins triggered by declining levels of estrogen and progesterone just before the onset of menstruation.

Epinephrine: one of two "stress" hormones secreted by the adrenal glands that acts as a powerful stimulant, increasing breathing, heart, and metabolic rates, constricting blood vessels and strengthening muscle contraction.

Estrogen: a hormone produced by the ovaries that helps thicken the uterine lining in preparation for pregnancy.

Evening primrose oil: a nutritional supplement that contains *gamma linoleic acid*, a saturated fatty acid necessary for the manufacture of certain prostaglandins in the body. The supplement is often sold in health food stores as a remedy for premenstrual symptoms. One study has suggested that evening primrose oil may reduce premenstrual breast tenderness, but there's no evidence that the nutritional supplement relieves other premenstrual symptoms.

Fight-or-flight response: a physiological response to a real or perceived physical or psychological stressor, in which the adrenal glands release the "stress" hormones epinephrine and norepinephrine, which accelerate breathing and pulse rate, raise blood pressure and blood sugar levels, and release stored fats into the bloodstream to provide the body with quick energy.

Follicle stimulating hormone: a hormone secreted by the pituitary gland in the brain that stimulates the growth of egg sacs (follicles) in the ovaries.

Follicular phase: the first half of a woman's menstrual cycle (beginning from the first day of menstruation), during which follicle stimulating hormone secreted by the pituitary gland in the brain stimulates the growth of several follicles (sacs containing germ cells that ripen into eggs) in the ovaries. The follicles in the ovaries, in turn, begin secreting estrogen.

GnRH agonists: these drugs block the secretion of gonadotropin releasing hormone by the hypothalamus, reducing the pituitary gland's secretion of follicle stimulating hormone and luteinizing hormone, and ultimately halting estrogen and progesterone production by the ovaries. The drugs have been found to be highly effective in relieving PMS among severely affected women. To avoid the menopause-related side effects of hot flashes and the potential risk of rapid bone loss associated with long term use of GnRH agonists, the drugs should be taken together with postmenopausal hormones (both estrogen and progestogen).

Gonadotropin releasing hormone (GnRH): a hormone released from the hypothalamus in the brain that stimulates the release of follicle stimulating hormone and luteinizing hormone (also known as gonadotropins) from the pituitary gland.

Hormones: chemical messengers that circulate in the bloodstream, stimulating or suppressing the actions of other glands or tissues in the body.

Hypoglycemia: lower than normal blood sugar levels (less than 50 milligrams per deciliter of blood), usually caused by a poor diet or by over-administration of insulin among people with diabetes. Symptoms include headache, weakness, irritability, and personality changes. Since many of the symptoms mimic those of PMS, scientists have suspected that women with PMS are actually suffering hypoglycemic episodes. So far, there's little evidence to support this theory.

Hypothalamus: part of the brain that controls the endocrine (glandular) system and such bodily functions as temperature regulation, hunger, thirst, and the development of secondary sex characteristics. The hypothalamus also governs certain strong emotions, notably anger. Among the hormones secreted by the hypothalamus is gonadotropin releasing hormone (GnRH), which signals the pituitary gland to produce follicle stimulating hormone and luteinizing hormone, hormones that help orchestrate women's menstrual cycles.

Hysterectomy with bilateral salpingo-oophorectomy: surgical removal of the uterus, both fallopian tubes, and both ovaries.

Hysterectomy: surgical removal of the uterus; the ovaries and fallopian tubes remain intact. This operation is sometimes referred to as a simple hysterectomy.

Inhibin: a hormone produced by the ovaries that helps signal the pituitary gland to stop secreting follicle stimulating hormone and *luteinizing hormone*.

L-tryptophan: see *Tryptophan*.

Late luteal phase dystrophic disorder (LLPDD): the name listed in the appendix of the Diagnostic and Statistical Manual of Mental Disorders, third edition (DSM-III, the diagnostic "bible" of psychiatrists) that is used to describe a subset of women with premenstrual syndrome whose dominant symptoms are related to mood disturbances. The category was added to the DSM-III in 1985 as a "diagnostic category needing further study," a move that was meant to facilitate more rigorous clinical research of the syndrome. Professionals often use the term interchangeably with premenstrual syndrome.

Leukotrienes: substances formed from arachidonic acid (a fatty acid in meat and dairy products) that regulate allergic and inflammatory reactions in the body. Some researchers believe these compounds may contribute to breast tenderness and other physical discomforts associated with PMS.

Luteal phase: the second half of a woman's menstrual cycle (beginning on day 14 of a 28-day cycle), during which the hormone progesterone is secreted from the corpus luteum, the empty egg sac in the ovary from which a ripe egg was released. Most symptoms associated with premenstrual syndrome occur late in the luteal phase of the menstrual cycle.

Luteinizing hormone: a hormone secreted by the pituitary gland in the brain that stimulates the ripening and release of an egg from the ovaries.

Magnesium: an essential mineral that plays a role in the body's manufacture of the neurotransmitter dopamine, secretion of the hormone insulin (which regulates blood-sugar levels), the manufacture of prostaglandins and the production of aldosterone. There's evidence to suggest that women with PMS have a magnesium deficiency, and that magnesium supplements help relieve premenstrual symptoms.

Mastalgia: the medical term for breast tenderness and swelling.

Melatonin: a hormone secreted only at night by the pineal gland in the brain. The hormone can be used as a marker of the body's biological clock. Women with PMS have been found to have lower levels of melatonin during the luteal phase of the menstrual cycle, suggesting that premenstrual symptoms in some women may be related to desynchronization of the body's biological clock.

Menarche: a woman's first menstrual period, usually occurring between the ages of nine and sixteen.

Menorrhagia: abnormally heavy or prolonged menstrual periods.

Menstrual migraine: severe headaches often accompanied by nausea, vomiting, and sensitivity to light or sound that occur only during the week before or the week of menstruation. These headaches are believed to be caused by fluctuating estrogen levels during the menstrual cycle.

Menstruation: the monthly shedding of the uterine lining (endometrium) when pregnancy doesn't occur.

Methylxanthines: chemicals in coffee, tea, cocoa, caffeine-containing colas and other soft drinks, and chocolates. Excessive consumption of these chemicals is suspected of exacerbating breast tenderness associated with premenstrual syndrome.

Neurotransmitters: chemicals released from nerve endings that enable nerve impulses to travel from one nerve cell to another in the brain and in other parts of the body. Common neurotransmitters are serotonin, dopamine and norepinephrine. An imbalance of neurotransmitters, particularly serotonin and dopamine, has been associated with depression and other emotional disorders.

Norepinephrine: one of two "stress" hormones secreted by the adrenal glands that constrict small blood vessels, raise blood pressure, slow the heart rate and increase the rate of breathing. The chemical is also one of several neurotransmitters released from nerve endings in the brain and other parts of the body.

Oophorectomy: surgical removal of one or both ovaries. Also known as *ovariectomy*.

Oral micronized progesterone: a natural progesterone (as opposed to the synthetic progestogens in oral contraceptives) in the form of a pill that is sometimes used to treat anxiety and other premenstrual symptoms.

Ovariectomy: surgical removal of one or both ovaries. Also known as *oophorectomy*.

Ovary: one of two sex organs located in a woman's abdomen that contain hundreds of thousands of germ cells, each encased in a sac of cells known as a follicle. Each month, under the influence of follicle stimulating hormone and luteinizing hormone secreted by the pituitary gland, one of the ovaries releases a mature egg, a process known as ovulation. Throughout the menstrual cycle, the ovaries secrete various amounts of the hormones estrogen, progesterone, testosterone, and inhibin.

Ovulation: the monthly release of an egg by the ovaries.

Placebo response: a phenomenon in which a patient's anticipation that a particular treatment will work are so high that even a sugar pill relieves symptoms.

Premenstrual syndrome: a cluster of symptoms, including water retention, breast tenderness, mood swings, irritability and depression, which generally worsen during the week or two before menstruation among women of reproductive age, then disappear altogether within one or two days of the start of menstruation.

Progesterone: a hormone produced by the ovaries after ovulation that helps thicken the uterine lining in preparation for pregnancy.

Prolactin: a hormone secreted by the pituitary gland that is involved in the development of the breasts at puberty and in breast milk production. The hormone is suspected of causing premenstrual breast tenderness.

Propranolol (Inderal): an antihypertensive drug sometimes prescribed to help prevent menstrual migraines.

Prostaglandin inhibitors: a class of drugs that relieves pain and other physical discomforts by blocking the production of prostaglandins in the body. Prostaglandin inhibitors commonly used in the treatment of PMS include ibuprofen (Motrin, Advil), mefenamic acid (Ponstel) and naproxen (Anaprox). These drugs are also known as nonsteroidal anti-inflammatory agents.

Prostaglandins: substances produced in such tissues as the brain, breasts, gastrointestinal tract, kidney, and reproductive tract, which have wide-ranging effects, influencing the capillaries, the nervous and endocrine (hormonal) systems, and smooth muscle. Over-production of prostaglandins by the uterus is associated with painful periods (dysmenorrhea) and an imbalance of prostaglandins has long been suspected of causing a variety of premenstrual symptoms.

Pyridoxine: see *Vitamin B₆*.

Renin: an enzyme released by the kidneys that converts biologically inactive angiotensin in the blood into an active form, helping to maintain the body's sodium and fluid balance.

Seasonal affective disorder: a type of depression that is linked with the change of seasons and daylight hours during the year. Sufferers usually experience depression, increased appetite, and carbohydrate cravings during the winter months, when daylight hours are shorter. The disorder is believed to be caused by a desynchronization of the body's biological clock. Bright light therapy—exposing patients to bright lights for several hours—has been found to help reset the biological clocks of affected people and alleviate depression. Researchers, noting similarities between seasonal affective disorder and PMS, have begun looking into whether the biological clocks of women with PMS are also somehow disturbed.

Sensory neuropathy: a type of nerve damage that sometimes occurs among women taking high levels (usually more than 200 mg per day) of vitamin B$_6$ for several months. Symptoms include burning, shooting, or tingling sensations in the hands and feet, clumsiness, and an unsteady gait. Symptoms clear up gradually after vitamin B$_6$ use is discontinued.

Serotonin: one of several neurotransmitters in the brain that allow nerve cells to communicate with one another. Low levels of serotonin are associated with depression.

Sodium: a mineral that is the main component of table salt. In the body, sodium helps maintain blood volume and fluid balance, helps transport nutrients and waste materials across cell walls, and aids in the transmission of nerve impulses. A high sodium diet may encourage fluid retention (edema) in the body's tissues.

Spironolactone (Aldactone): a potassium-sparing diuretic often prescribed to relieve bloating and fluid retention associated with premenstrual syndrome. The drug works by blocking the water-retaining action of the hormone aldosterone.

Tamoxifen (Nolvadex): a drug commonly used in the treatment of postmenopausal women with estrogen-dependent breast cancer. The drug is sometimes prescribed to relieve breast tenderness associated with premenstrual syndrome.

Total hysterectomy: surgical removal of the uterus and the cervix (opening of the uterus). The ovaries remain intact. See also, Hysterectomy with bilateral salpingo-oophorectomy.

Tryptophan: an amino acid that is converted into the neurotransmitter serotonin in the brain. L-tryptophan, a nutritional supplement once sold as a sleep aid and treatment for premenstrual syndrome, was banned in 1990 by the United States Food and Drug Administration after a contaminated batch of supplements manufactured in Japan was associated with a rare, potentially life-threatening blood disorder known as eosinophilia myalgia syndrome.

Uterus: the thick-walled muscular cavity within a women's pelvis that nourishes a growing fetus during pregnancy. The uterus consists of three layers: an inner mucus layer, known as the endometrium, which sheds and bleeds during menstruation and nourishes the growing fetus during pregnancy; a muscular layer known as the myometrium which, during labor and childbirth, contracts to help push the baby out; and the parametrium, an outer layer of connective tissues.

Vitamin B$_6$: also known as pyridoxine. This water soluble vitamin, found in such foods as yeast, wheat germ, sunflower seeds, chicken, tuna, legumes, whole grain cereals, bananas, and oatmeal, is instrumental in the body's manufacture of the neurotransmitter serotonin. A deficiency of vitamin B$_6$ is associated with depression. High doses of vitamin B$_6$ may cause sensory neuropathy, a type of nerve damage that causes such symptoms as shooting or tingling pains and numbness in the hands and feet, clumsiness or an unsteady gait.

Vitamin E: a fat-soluble vitamin (also known as tocopherol) believed to be involved in the production of certain prostaglandins and leukotrienes. Vitamin E supplements are often recommended for the relief of breast tenderness associated with premenstrual syndrome.

INDEX

ABOUT THE AUTHORS

ANDREA J. RAPKIN, M.D., F.A.C.O.G., an Associate Professor at the UCLA School of Medicine, has extensive clinical experience and is a reviewer for several prominent medical journals, including the *American Journal of Obstetrics and Gynecology*. She is an active researcher in the field of PMS.

DIANA TONNESSEN, a freelance writer and former managing editor for *Health* magazine, has written articles for *American Baby*, *McCall's*, and *Self*. She is also the co-author (with Morris Notelovitz, M.D., Ph.D.) of *Menopause and Midlife Health*.